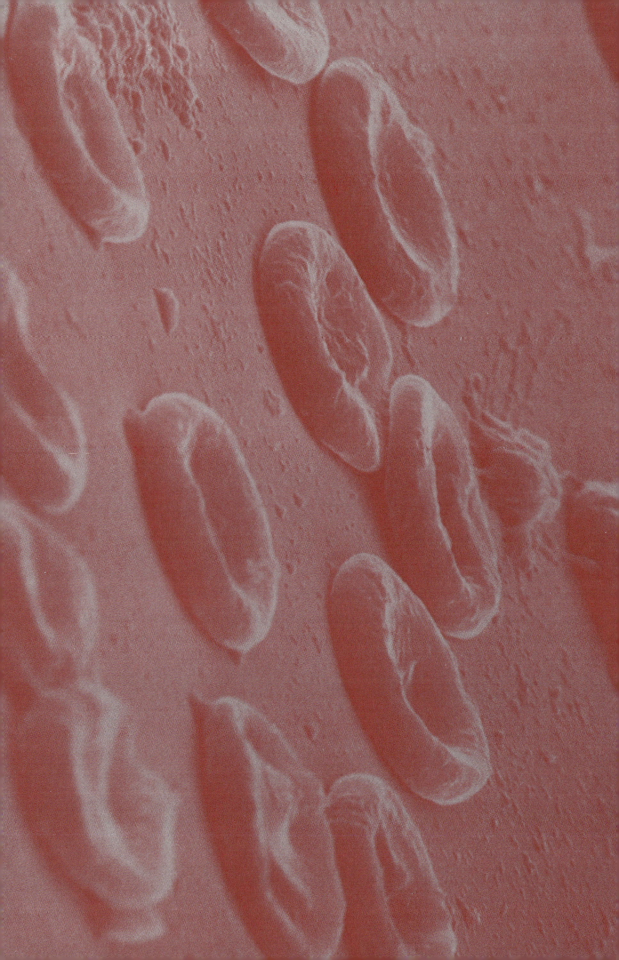

LEARNING FOR OUR COMMON HEALTH

HOW AN ACADEMIC FOCUS ON HIV/AIDS WILL IMPROVE EDUCATION AND HEALTH

Wm. David Burns, Editor

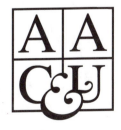

ASSOCIATION OF AMERICAN COLLEGES AND UNIVERSITIES
WASHINGTON, DC

Published by the
Association of American Colleges and Universities,
1818 R Street NW, Washington, DC 20009

Copyright 1999

This publication was produced by the Program for Health and Higher Education with support provided under a cooperative agreement (Number U87/CCU312248) with the U.S. Centers for Disease
Control and Prevention, National Center for Chronic Disease Prevention and Health Promotion,
Division of Adolescent and School Health, Atlanta, Georgia. Its contents are solely the responsibility
of the authors and do not necessarily represent the official views of U.S. Centers for Disease Control
and Prevention.

ISBN 0-011696-76-8

Published by the
Association of American Colleges and Universities,
1818 R Street NW, Washington, DC 20009

This publication was produced by the Program for Health and Higher Education with support provided under a cooperative agreement (Number U87/CCU312248) with the U.S. Centers for Disease Control and Prevention, National Center for Chronic Disease Prevention and Health Promotion, Division of Adolescent and School Health, Atlanta, Georgia. Its contents are solely the responsibility of the authors and do not necessarily represent the official views of U.S. Centers for Disease Control and Prevention.

ISBN 0-011696-76-8

LEARNING FOR OUR COMMON HEALTH

HOW AN ACADEMIC FOCUS ON HIV/AIDS WILL IMPROVE EDUCATION AND HEALTH

Wm. David Burns, Editor

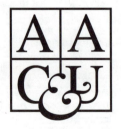

ASSOCIATION OF AMERICAN COLLEGES AND UNIVERSITIES
WASHINGTON, DC

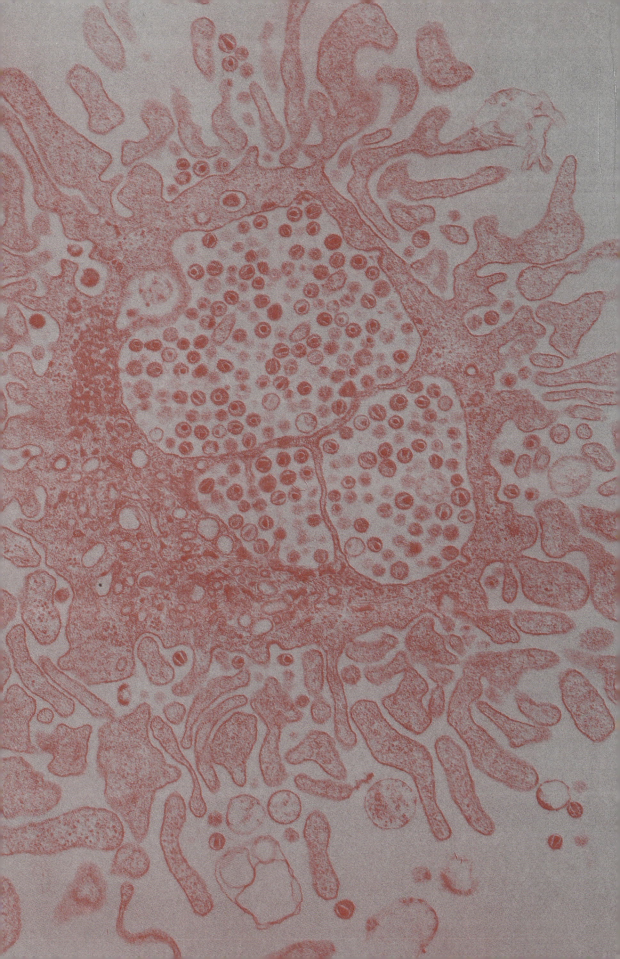

ONE

LEARNING FOR OUR COMMON HEALTH

Wm. David Burns

ASSOCIATION OF AMERICAN COLLEGES AND UNIVERSITIES

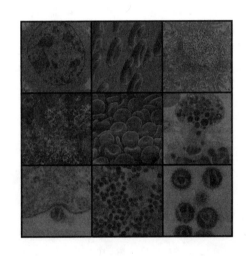

To students and faculty members, and especially to our Partners in Health and Higher Education, across the nation:

Students and teachers learning together in classrooms, laboratories, and in their communities all around the country are among the many intended beneficiaries of this work. They are also the people who have made the work possible, through their interest and experience in bringing the issues health and HIV/AIDS in particular into undergraduate education. Our work and thinking at AAC&U has also been particularly influenced by our project partners who have been developing, testing, and refining strategies to improve education and health. (The partnership institutions are named in the Resource section of this book.)

To Ms. K. Mary Hess and Bristol-Myers Squibb:

Distribution of this book was made possible, in part, from an unrestricted grant from Bristol-Myers Squibb that supplemented funds available for production and distribution. This support means that the book will reach many more leaders in higher education and public health and that copies will be available for use on campus. Special appreciation is due Ms. K. Mary Hess, who was instrumental in securing this support from her company.

The authors of these essays are responsible for their own work. As the editor, I have tried to take a very light hand, privileging the strength of each author's analyses, arguments, and convictions over a forced consistency or unity for the book as a whole. Hence, there is some redundancy, and, quite naturally, not all the authors would agree with all that others are arguing. Some of the authors do, however, seem to be speaking to one another, conscious of their engagement in this collective work. Others do not display this consciousness, due in part to the fact that the pieces were written and collected over a period of almost three years; this fact also accounts for the modest absence of synchronicity among the pieces.

Readers are invited to hold me responsible for the overall conception of this book and for any lapses in gracefulness or other by-products of what we tried to make ensemble rather than solo work.

Wm. David Burns
Washington, 1999

our work at Rutgers University that led up to this project, as well.

To the National Leadership Advisory Board of the Program for Health and Higher Education:

Our project has been blessed by the constant support of and wise counsel from a distinguished group of leaders (whose names are printed in this book) who have guided the project, volunteered their labor to help achieve project goals, written and adopted a national leadership statement (also printed in this book), reviewed materials and, authored several of the essays in this book. One could not hope for more from a Board. Special recognition is also due to NLAB member, Dr. Richard Keeling, who has served as a senior scholar on this project since its inception and whose influence over our work is immeasurable.

To colleagues at the Association of American Colleges and Universities:

Special thanks are due to our past president, Paula Brownlee, who saw the need for this work within the larger effort to improve undergraduate education, and to our current president, Carol Geary Schneider, whose wise guidance is discernible throughout this monograph, including its title, which she suggested. Other colleagues meriting special mention are: Robert Shoenberg, AAC&U senior scholar and evaluation consultant to PHHE; Joann Stevens, vice president for communications and a member of the PHHE project team; Bridget Puzon, senior editor and editor of *Liberal Education* (where several of these essays have already appeared); Diane Knich, PHHE project associate; and Rafael Heller, assistant editor. Other colleagues who have made specific and long-term contributions to PHHE's work include Eliza Reilly, Tony Wiggins, and Suzanne Hyers. Special mention must also be made of and thanks expressed to Dr. William O'Connell, who, while a visiting fellow at AAC&U in 1995-96, helped us attract the interest of higher education leaders to this effort. This is an incomplete list, to say the least, because it is no exaggeration to say that we at AAC&U are a small enough team to each benefit from the large and diverse set of talents and expertise available to us.

To the people who made this book:

The "look" of this book represents the talents of its designer, Steven Nathaniel Nutter, and Michael Nottingham, who carried the production of this book to completion. Both worked hard to produce these results.

ACKNOWLEDGMENTS

Simple, direct and sincere thanks are due and tendered to the following people, without whom this book would not exist:

To our authors: Nora Bell, Robert Corrigan, William Cronon, Mindy Thompson Fullilove, Robert Fullilove, Ira Harkavy, Richard Keeling, Sheila McClear, Patsy Reed, and Daniel Romer.

This book is the product of the work of many contributing authors, so it is to them that the largest debt of gratitude is owed. Throughout the period in which we commissioned and collected the following essays, the authors worked diligently, sometimes under very tight deadlines, often within newly developing conceptions of what we hoped to accomplish with this text. Through it all, they were conscientious and almost always cheerful. In part, I suspect, this springs from their sincere interest in helping others to become engaged in this work and expresses their own deep commitments to improving education and health. Profoundly humanitarian in their approaches, our authors are the very models of citizens willing to place their energies and intelligence in the service of improving the human condition.

To our colleagues at Department of Health and Human Services—US Centers for Disease Control and Prevention: David Satcher, James Marks, Helene Gayle, Lloyd Kolbe, Diane Allensworth, Gloria Bryan, and Dean Fenley.

The Program for Health and Higher Education (PHHE) would not exist but for the support of the US Centers for Disease Control and Prevention, and the individuals mentioned here. Lloyd Kolbe, the director of the Division of Adolescent and School Health, had the singular insight that it would take schools and colleges and universities—and not just public health departments—working collaboratively to improve the health of young people. With that insight came the development of a series of programs to engage leaders from several sectors in efforts to reduce disease and improve health. Bringing these issues into the undergraduate education of students —into what it means to be educated—is another advance that could not have happened without Dr. Satcher's, Dr. Marks' and Dr. Gayle's support. In addition to that general support, I want to acknowledge the specific contributions of Lloyd Kolbe to our thinking, and to express appreciation to Diane Allensworth, Gloria Bryan and Dean Fenley for their advice and help over the years of this project, and, in the case of Diane and Dean, in

On behalf of its 700 institutional members representing some four million students, AAC&U extends a special thanks to the United States Centers for Disease Control and Prevention (CDC) for sponsoring this significant initiative and giving us the opportunity to work with higher education leaders and the nation in this very important area of public health. We are privileged to be able to assist leaders who share our greater expectations for improving learning and making a difference in our nation's health and well being.

Carol Geary Schneider
President
Association of American Colleges and Universities

FOREWORD

Four years ago, the Association of American Colleges and Universities' Program for Health and Higher Education (PHHE) launched a bold model to help leaders improve undergraduate learning by engaging higher education in the solution to one of the world's most pressing problems: preventing HIV disease and reducing the threat it poses to youth. PHHE recognized the issue as a complex social problem and located its relevance within the academic mission of the academy. In so doing, PHHE helped leaders inspire a new generation of students to explore this important personal and public issue through the capacious and creative lens of liberal learning. Biology, literature, economics, ethics, the sociology of race, class and health, history and women's studies became just a few of the entry points through which science and non-science majors were invited to consider the "multidisciplinary trouble" of HIV/AIDS.

Responding to needs identified by campus leaders, faculty development seminars and conferences have introduced scores of PHHE participants to new learning strategies, interactive technology, curricular innovations, and service learning models about HIV/AIDS and health, all within the context of powerful new pedagogies and important educational reforms. Model projects were selected and have been supported at twenty-seven campuses. An interactive, searchable national leadership resource database is currently under development. A statement on *HIV, Health and Higher Education* that was adopted by AAC&U's board of directors locates these efforts within the context of educational mission.

Now we are proud to release this monograph that reflects the lessons learned and insights gained from the PHHE initiative, while describing new questions being pondered by leaders of higher education and public health. The voices and experiences of some of the nation's leading educational and health authorities who have engaged with PHHE resound forcefully from this monograph. The authors explore the case for this new scholarship; for re-thinking how we conceptualize health, and for using common health to improve the capacity of our students to be active participants in our democratic society. They also suggest approaches that connect knowledge to personal action in responsible ways. In considering how and why an academic focus on HIV/AIDS can improve learning and our common health, the monograph makes a compelling case. Its essays will contribute to achieving a broad range of campus and community goals.

CONTENTS

The Association of American Colleges and Universities' (AAC&U) Program for Health and Higher Education (PHHE) centers on a complex social problem, framed within a simple, powerful approach. We ask: If higher education would place a strong, academic focus on a problem—such as HIV and health—would the end result advance our greater expectations for student learning, academic rigor, faculty authority, collaborative leadership, social responsibility, and civic engagement? Moreover, would such a strong academic focus lead to solutions to the complex problem itself? In a word, we think the answer is "yes."

The purpose of this monograph is to explore these questions and to consider how and why an academic focus on HIV/AIDS can improve learning and our common health. The essays collected here encourage and justify such academic attention by connecting it to the best principles of academic practice. While the essays are foundational in nature, they also suggest strategies designed to help academic leaders achieve good results.

This opening essay serves as an introduction to the book, providing a broad conceptual framework for considering the issues raised and arguments made by our authors. As the director of the PHHE project and the editor of the present collection, I explain the approach we are taking, discuss the two complementary strands of our thinking, suggest how learning might help inform personal choices and behavior, consider important challenges to innovation and change, and, in the context of the fight for our students' bodies, urge attention to our common health. Finally, the essay provides a map introducing our contributors and suggesting where their essays are located within this larger project. A set of suggestions for using these essays—with a variety of campus constituencies and in connection with a similarly broad collection of campus purposes—is provided in the resources section at the very end of the book.

WHAT WE LEARNED FROM LISTENING TO LEADERS

We began our project by listening to what leaders had to say about both the desirability of bringing the study of HIV into the classroom as well as the utility of doing so. We wanted to know if leaders thought this approach was a good idea. And from those who did, we wanted to know what benefits such an approach could bring. What did leaders need from us?

What we learned encouraged us and pointed out the need for a monograph that would develop the "theory" for this work. On a practical level, leaders asked for models. That spurred us to develop our partnership program, which has to date supported pilot projects at twenty-six institutions. These two findings will illustrate just a small part of what we learned:

- More than 70 percent of the presidents and chief academic officers who responded to our surveys (and more than 800 did, representing almost 4 million students) told us that such academic inclusion was "very important" or "essential." Fewer reported that such inclusion was already under way. Thus, many were inclined to support new efforts in this direction on their campuses.

- On the questions about the usefulness (or ends) of such study, about two-thirds of the chief academic officers responding agreed that the inclusion of HIV/AIDS inquiry in the classroom had especially significant potential for achieving a number of important academic and civic goals. These included: helping students face issues they must face, raising issues of ethics and moral responsibility, understanding public policy issues, integrating academic and student life goals, engaging the interest of non-science majors in science, understanding diversity issues, and improving public health (Burns 1997).

We received broad general support and a reservoir of good will about the aims of the project. Beyond that, we were told our help was needed.

TRANSLATING GENERAL SUPPORT INTO PLANS FOR IMPROVEMENT

Broad support for a concept is very different from agreement about the nature and extent of what should be done, or who should do it, or what results might really be predicted if it is done, or for that matter, why it should be done. So, even with the general support, we felt an obligation to provide a foundation and rationale for using health and HIV/AIDS to improve learning. We also needed to justify the *use* of higher education to focus on health in a general way. In addition, we felt compelled to explore how what we hoped leaders would support is connected to other traditions and reforms in higher education. To do this, we asked several academic leaders and scholars to help us explore and expand this idea.

Our authors were not just operating theoretically. Readers will see that all are working from direct experience in a variety of leadership, faculty, and administrative roles. And, as scholars, they are also speaking as students, for they are reporting on what they have learned and are learning, as well. I draw on their work in this essay.

This monograph advocates several innovations and improvements in education generally as well as the consideration of health in education, specifically. As authors we share several other goals, joining all those who desire:

- to reduce the spread of HIV, improve health, and eliminate the terrible disparities in health outcomes that affect our citizens—disparities that are, as often as not, related to unresolved issues of race and gender;

- to help students examine their own personal beliefs and behavior and to strengthen our students' sense of responsibility to themselves and to others;

- to improve intellectual development and expand knowledge; and

- to increase the capacity of graduates to be active and effective civic and moral agents, exercising their responsibilities in the world of work, in the civic arena, and in their personal lives.

Taken together, these essays suggest how we might think about health and how thinking about health would help us to think better, generally. Reciprocally, all suggest that improved thinking and learning is a fundamental pre-condition for the general improvement of health.

TWO COMPLEMENTARY FOUNDATIONS, ONE NEW APPROACH

In this monograph many of the arguments take a form resembling the double helix— that is, two strands that wind around each other—or like those wonderful bronze ramps in the entry to the Vatican Museums, or the elaborate double circular "communicating" staircases found in some tall monuments, where some are climbing on one set of steps while, on another set, others are descending around them.

There are two strands to our work:

An academic focus on HIV and health, as a complex, multi-dimensional public problem of great consequence, has the capacity to improve undergraduate education. Let's start with our own core academic mission, namely guaranteeing the integrity, rigor, quality, and effectiveness of the education we offer and the learning and knowledge we expect that it will produce. Above all, we in higher education are responsible for achieving this mission.

Within this mission, our argument—and that of many commentators—is that such learning will be improved through the employment of complex, pressing problems that are capacious. That is, the problems should be capacious enough in their nature so as to require the application of a broad range of disciplinary perspectives and traditions in order to establish meanings (make sense of the issue), to explain their workings (understand the dynamics of the issue), and to fashion effective strategies to limit or increase their power or saliency (affect the issue). These kinds of issues, themes, or questions will require learning that is active and connected. They may demand newly designed research initiatives and approaches, just as they will make use of the products of past research efforts. And, where human behavior is involved—and where is it not?—the effective consideration of these problems and issues will benefit from an understanding of human nature, an appreciation for human commonalities and differences, and, in our context, a good grasp of the democratic processes (the arts of citizenship) required to deliberate and achieve effective consideration in the public sphere.

The best candidates for this kind of study will be contested, unresolved issues whose outcome is not yet certain. Students should actually be working on their resolution. If the issues engage student interests and if students perceive that they have some stake in them, then student engagement will be more vibrant.

Most important, good organizing themes and problems will require not just the consumption of knowledge or the acquisition of a technique or skill, but the development and production of new knowledge and the refinement of existing techniques and skills, or perhaps even the invention of new ones.

Ideally, these themes or organizing strategies for education should also contain doorways and passageways to the insights of the past. The critique, if any, of what has gone before should serve, at least to some degree, to suggest the uncertainty and provisional nature of what is thought to be known at this moment. The sensitive and rigorous consideration of these issues should help cultivate habits of mind—like discernment and inquisitiveness—as well as encourage a disposition to both think for oneself and act with broader consequences in mind.

We submit that HIV/AIDS, in particular, and the whole complex set of things that we mean when we say health, meet these criteria and serve these ends well. Other topics do, as well, although few require as many of the broad range of assets that good colleges and universities have to offer. As our authors demonstrate, and Professor Cronon asserts, "AIDS in fact connects to almost everything."

The assets of a good undergraduate education, properly directed, have the capacity to improve health and decrease the spread of the HIV. To those—like the CDC—whose core mission is to try to improve the nation's health, reduce the incidence of HIV infection, and better manage the infection so as to improve the lives of those affected, the needs for connection to higher education can be argued for and demonstrated in several ways.

First, of course, those engaged in prevention, treatment, and management require the assets that are represented in higher education's enormous capacity and accomplishment in the production of knowledge. From research laboratories, whose scholars are engaged in basic research, to laboratory schools, where theory and practice inform one another every day; the intellectual power residing in higher education is fundamental to the nation's and the world's efforts to discover the causes and cures for diseases and to explain how people can be engaged, individually and collectively, in the improvement of their own lives and the lives of others.

The resources of higher education are also of enormous value in three other specific areas as well:

1. the development and analysis of public policy (helping to answer a range of questions that fall under the general question of "What should political entities do about health?");

2. the evaluation of efforts undertaken (helping to answer a range of questions whose general form is "What works and what doesn't?"); and,

3. the ongoing (in-service) education of those who are engaged in health work so as to ensure that they have the benefits of the latest and best thinking to put in the service of their practice. These functions serve broad community needs. They are externally directed.

Internally, there are two significant reasons why those charged with improving the nation's health should turn to undergraduate education, especially in regard to HIV/AIDS:

1. *Colleges and universities have large cohorts of individuals whose behavior exposes them to specific risks and who are "reachable" and thus, perhaps, teachable.* Like much late adolescent and early adult behavior, student behavior describes a series of patterns that create opportunities for, and in many instances actually predict, acute and chronic health risks. While there is debate about the "infiltration" of HIV/AIDS in the general student body (see Dr. Keeling's essay), there is little disagreement about its potential for devastating consequences. Were HIV to be introduced in certain circles of sexual encounters, the results could soon become dire. It would be too grandiose a claim to say that the current attention to prevention accounts for this apparent failure of HIV to explode in the student population, especially since the evidence of behavior change is only slightly encouraging. But, without such evidence, the opportunity and conditions are present for the expansion of HIV and other epidemics that are nurtured by certain sexual encounters and the

exchange of blood. Dr. Keeling, as well as Dr. Corrigan and Ms. McClear, are also quite clear in their assessment that alcohol misuse and abuse—a major health problem on campuses—are significant co-factors whose connection to the potential spread of HIV is especially significant. So this is not just an argument for paying special attention where it is due; it is also an argument about convenience and efficiency—as people (students) at special risk can be reached effectively and with relative ease.

2. *Colleges and universities are responsible for the education of most of the professionals who will be affecting prevention and health care delivery, as well as the education of those who will be leaders in a variety of professions whose work can contribute to or detract from the nation's and the world's health. Colleges are also engaged in the important work of educating citizens.* Regardless of whether any one particular student will contract HIV/AIDS (and it appears right now that most will not), a huge cohort of our graduates will enter fields where they will be called upon to have an understanding of HIV/AIDS. And all but a very few have, or will soon have, civic and family roles where engagement with the many issues raised by HIV/AIDS and other "diseases of new encounters" will be not only useful, but in many cases, essential.

Given the fact that HIV/AIDS is increasingly being described as a disease of those who are not receiving the benefits and privileges of a higher education, the consideration of this epidemic—not just in terms of private risk but also of public obligation—may be a necessary precondition for its effective treatment in the public sphere, where decisions about policies and resources will be made.

In summary, it would be fair to conclude that our project urges two kinds of "opportunism." First, we suggest that HIV/AIDS be used, instrumentally, to improve learning. Second, we say that learning (undergraduate, classroom, laboratory, and field-based academic work, linked, where appropriate, to specific prevention efforts that are generally developed and delivered by student life personnel and peer educators) should be used both to improve student health and prepare graduates to improve our common health.

THE FIGHT FOR OUR STUDENTS' BODIES (AND THEIR ATTENTION AS WELL)

Before we can effectively consider how the approach we advocate would work, it would be useful to consider just how much attention is now given to our students' bodies. To begin, Alfred North Whitehead's injunction to remember the body, written

more than seventy-five years ago, is worth repeating. In the essay "The Aims of Education," Whitehead (1961) wrote:

> I lay it down as an educational axiom that in teaching you will come to grief as soon as you forget that your pupils have bodies. This is exactly the mistake of the post-renaissance Platonic curriculum. But nature can be kept at bay with no pitchfork.

This view bears repeating because, given our bias towards the mind and its development, we all too often fail to observe the great competition for our students' bodies. This competition is really about the mind, of course, but it hides itself in the form of attention to the body and body image, and exploits a realm of feelings, sensations, and images.

The competition for students' bodies has dramatic and far-reaching dimensions beyond those that would touch on traditional conceptions of health. And, as commerce, what a competition it is! Students are an important market for all kinds of things from alcohol, clothes, vacations, cars, and credit cards to concerts, coiffures, and CDs; from perfumes to piercings. My own conservative estimate of the value of this "market"—assuming a modest average of $30 per week expenditure for a host of consumables beyond food, shelter, and education—produces an annual target worth more than $11 billion a year. That's part of the "context" to be faced by those who would try to influence these minds and the bodies that come to college with them.

But the fight for the body is only one struggle. The competition for attention is at least as fierce; attention to academic performance vies with the demands for attention from employment, family and friends, partners, roommates, fellow team members, TV, the Internet, the telephone, and on and on. Kenneth Gergen's (1991) description of the "saturated self" expresses this idea effectively. This saturation has consequences for educators generally, and particularly for those who are trying to stir up interest during the time students are not in class.

We have observed that most leaders support HIV/AIDS education and the academically based approach we advocate. Most students, however, seem to have concluded that HIV is not a significant personal risk or issue. Surely there are significant exceptions to this, but as Dr. Corrigan and Ms. McClear at San Francisco State University report in their essay, even San Francisco State University faces a challenge attracting and holding student attention. This lack of interest is also reported by Dr. Keeling.

Given the competition for students' attention, such "apathy" is understandable, especially when we consider the way a great deal of prevention education is presented and how important students think this education is to them personally. As often as not, prevention education is presented as a product or "program" to be consumed,

whether in the form of a pamphlet, film, exhibition, celebrity lecture, the designation of an "AIDS" day, or one "stop" for STDs along the long orientation road. Much of the prevention education itself begins in an individual assessment of risk leading to an immediate disconnect, because to many students HIV/AIDS currently does not seem like a big risk ("my friends don't have it"). Unlike a few years ago, when "scare tactics" could be backed up with "facts," today, as a risk, HIV's most devastating medical consequences are *deferred*; that is, they don't happen right away. Further, given new treatments, HIV no longer seems to presage the "sure and quick death" that it once did. And, as the evidence suggests, increasingly, for white, heterosexual college students, HIV does seem to be exclusively a problem of "others."

Providing traditional HIV education currently is a challenge on campus. So, it is *not* surprising that health educators, working at the edge of the academy, have had to rely on students' good will and the use of "premiums" (and other gimmicks) to attract student attention.

Indeed, the strategies of social marketing that are being applied to traditional prevention methods are themselves devices to locate sales and service within more successful approaches aimed at influencing behavior, for good or bad ends. The weaknesses of our current approach have led many of our authors to advocate moving from consumption models to models of work and engagement. Dr. Keeling expresses this by urging a relocation of HIV/AIDS education from "the margin to the mission."

FROM "I" TO "EYE" AND BACK TO "ME": HOW WOULD THIS WORK?

Here's a sketch of how an academic consideration of HIV/AIDS might improve an individual's own capacity to act to reduce the risk of HIV. The strategy implied here is this:

1. *Begin with the self:* Start by assuming self-interest, self-assessment, and some consciousness of risk. Examine perceptions. Help discover assets (knowledge, experience, connections, capacities). Determine which qualities and habits of mind and individual capacities could be strengthened.

2. *Move beyond the self:* Engage in a broad consideration of what we mean by health and disease; explore the many contexts, the many meanings and the many explanations for human behavior. Apply the range of intellectual assets and practical experiential learning to the academic situation. Consider how differently claims about truth are heard and applied. Explore and evaluate connections between things.

3. *Return to the self:* Now think of one's self as a civic agent, moral actor, and life-long learner: What was learned on this tour or journey beyond the self? What was discovered that one needed to know? What capacity as a civic agent was developed? What personal, "selfish" changes now seem indicated? What is needed to connect knowledge and behavior?

4. *Repeat the process.*

This account is a bit crude, but readers will immediately recognize it as a model of production and development, and not an argument for the creation of a more effective ("new and improved") product to be consumed. Neither is it an argument for crude conformity. It leaves room for freedom—including the freedom to make mistakes—as a necessary dimension of education in a liberal democracy. Of course, it also provides a foundation for supporting particular prevention strategies and techniques available on campus and elsewhere. The approach also sets up a condition that can lead to improvement of these strategies and techniques, by welcoming the expression of particular needs, not pushing ready-made nostrums or advocating coercion. Fundamentally, this is an approach to learning that is especially and felicitously connected to a liberal education, to what Professor Cronon so eloquently calls "an education for human freedom."

CHALLENGES TO INNOVATION AND CHANGE

The arguments in this essay and this monograph will please those who accept the basic premise that one purpose of the academy is to help students learn to work out answers to large, unsolved, vexing questions that won't stay confined within traditional or existing disciplinary or other boundaries. The monograph will encourage those who think students should *produce*, not simply *consume* knowledge. It will also please those who think that one function of higher education is to put learning in the service of solving public problems, advancing common purposes with both integrity and commitment.

But the monograph is also produced out of respect for those who do not share these enthusiasms, or who have not thought about the issues extensively. It was written as well for those who have considered these issues carefully and who have principled objections to the kinds of innovations and approaches being advocated. We owe this examination to everyone, including those who would reject our conclusions. But we owe it especially to those whose attentions and energies we hope will be directed toward the dual purposes of improving education and health.

In this we are guided, in part, by the insights and analysis offered by Michael Oakeshott, the British political theorist, in his essay "On being conservative." There, Oakeshott (1991) makes the following points about innovation and change:

> [A]man of conservative temperament draws some appropriate conclusions. First, innovation entails certain loss and possible gain, therefore, the onus of proof, to show that the proposed change may be on the whole expected to be beneficial, rests on the would-be innovator. Secondly, he believes that the more closely the innovation resembles growth (that is, the more clearly it is intimated in and not merely imposed upon the situation) the less likely it is to result in a preponderance of loss. Thirdly, he thinks that an innovation which is in response to some specific defect, one designed to redress some specific disequilibrium, is more desirable than one that springs from a notion of generally improved condition of human circumstances, and is far more desirable than one generated by a vision of perfection. Fourthly, he favours a slow rather than a rapid pace, and pauses to observe current consequences and make appropriate adjustments. And lastly, he believes occasion to be important: and, all other things being equal, he considers the most favourable occasion for innovation to be when the projected change is most likely to be limited to what is intended and least likely to be corrupted by undesired and unmanageable consequences.

Oakeshott's cool rationality has always proved a tough test for those whose satisfaction with the status quo is, should we say, limited.

But what Oakeshott offers us, if we accept it, is a challenge, one that we have tried to incorporate in this work. We have done this first by suggesting how, for example, the focus on HIV/AIDS suits a general academic movement, one that grows from (or moves from) a strict disciplinary understanding to more general understandings of issues, including meta-issues like ethics, epistemology, pedagogy, and the complex question of the relationship of knowledge to action. Second, our focus is on shared, or common health (as opposed to focusing solely on individual risks) and on the disparities and efforts to redress current disequilibrium that may, among other things, locate health within too small a boundary, namely the individual human body and its biological processes. And this academic focus on "the body" addresses another disequilibrium that has long discounted the body in discussions or examinations of the mind. Third, our authors tend to advocate, as does Oakeshott, that observation is critical and that adjustments to respond to challenges are essential. (Consider how much of the Professors Fullilove's essay on race and "beliefs" corresponds with Oakeshott's notions of loss and onus.) The authors of the essays in this monograph may be visionaries, but they are not utopians.

In three areas, however, Oakeshott might find us wanting:

1. *pace*—The advocates of doing something to limit the disaster of HIV disease have indeed challenged the orderliness of many processes designed to achieve degrees of certainty, including academically inflected processes, like drug trials. In the world of HIV/AIDS—or any disease—many fools (with their lives at stake) have indeed rushed in where angels (with their reputations at stake) have feared to tread. Indeed, the pace we advocate might just displease everyone: those who think there is a crisis (and a good case can be made for that point of view) will not be satisfied with what can be a perceived as a calm, considered, take-the-long-view, developmental approach. And those who think that the academy should not sully itself with transient, contemporary crises of whatever nature or proportion will find even in baby-steps further evidence of our decline and fall.

    If we thought we had the "magic bullet," we would be rushing it public as well, but the fact that we have a strategy—one firmly grounded in traditions of good academic practice and not a product we want you to buy—suggests that implementation will be at a pace that might not entirely satisfy those who think urgency is required but will not alarm those inclined to err on the side of circumspection.

2. *occasion*—Surely the occasion for us to act is now. Nationally and worldwide we are deep into the epidemic; we know that a great deal of student behavior creates a constellation of risks that could result in catastrophic consequences when the disease organism enters a particular community; and we are involved in raising expectations to embrace substantial systemic reform to improve educational practice and achievement. But HIV/AIDS, and indeed any complex issue, is, by its nature, a little messier than Oakeshott might want it to be. Hence there is present not just the possibility but the likelihood that engagement with it will entail "undesired and unmanageable consequences." But you could say HIV/AIDS is already a bundle of such consequences. Many of our authors start their analyses with the observation by the distinguished former leader of the President's National Commission on AIDS, Dr. June Osborn, that "AIDS is multidisciplinary trouble." HIV/AIDS has been used already for many purposes, from advocating abstinence to supporting same-sex marriages (these do tend to originate in different parts of our political community). Part of the reason for rigorous academic consideration of HIV/AIDS isn't to add to the consequences, but to systematically examine them and sort them out.

3. *onus*—Indeed, the burden for us is to demonstrate—to accept Oakeshott's "onus"—that what we are proposing will, on the whole, be beneficial. In this case,

however, our challenge isn't that enormous, at least in Oakeshott's terms, because he proposes a kind of formula that suggests greater "onus" for changes that will produce greater "loss." What, if anything, would be lost in the effort to focus attention on HIV/AIDS in the classroom? What we are proposing will not, to use his terms again, entail "certain loss." Moreover, we cannot compel change. We employ no force other than the force of argument and—no small thing—an appeal to good results. But can we prove a benefit at this time? Surely, not as conclusively as we would like, but early results are encouraging. The published results of efforts so far have shown good academic outcomes, even when individual health outcomes were less than hoped for. The results achieved by our partners who are implementing these kinds of reform will help us demonstrate and determine outcomes. Above all, we are committed to knowing if the benefits justify the "certain loss" even while we seek to minimize any loss itself.

Let Oakeshott's analysis, however detached or unfeeling it may seem, inform us about the nature of change, not just the nature of change in the academy, but everywhere. His is surely not the only account of change we need to examine, but it is a good place to start as we try to find common cause to improve education and health. How then, might we think about "our common health"?

OUR COMMON HEALTH

It was about ten years ago at a meeting on health communication at the University of Kentucky that I first heard the words *common* and *health* used together to signify one idea. Sam Becker, distinguished professor at the University of Iowa, used "common health" to describe something broader than the idea of public health and larger than our idea of personal health. Expanding, or at least elevating, the idea of public health and exploring the limitations of too private a conception of health seemed to me a worthwhile project then. It still does today.

The attraction of the phrase "common health" has a different explanation, however. What appealed to me then and now is how "common" works in the phrase by really helping us to understand health in a new way. It helps the idea of health in much the same way as the addition of "common" helps in a variety of constructions I admire: common sense, common courtesy, common purpose, and in our own academic context, common core. The double meaning of "common" is appealing. Common suggests something on the one hand basic, ordinary, elemental, and pretty widely distributed, even ubiquitous. At the same time, however, it refers to a shared property, something held in common, collectively perhaps, but something that each of us has individually as well. Beyond this, common signifies connection and, thus, for me, implies both responsibility and reciprocity.

Common—in the sense of a communion open to all—helps us enter a space between a selfish and potentially cruel individualism or solipsism, on one side, and a liberty-crushing, "utopian" collectivism or mindless group-think, on the other. Of course, there lurk potentially dangerous assumptions in an unexamined "commonality" —indeed, some of the very same dangers that inhere in unexamined ideas of "difference." So this conception of health should carry a cautionary note—at least the academic equivalent of the Surgeon General's warning on a pack of cigarettes—that calls for further examination and exploration. This examination, ironically, will require uncommon knowledge and specialized approaches. It will also need to be tested against common knowledge and common experience.

Our modern, western ideas of health needed the tonic that Becker's modification "common" provided. Health sounds simple enough, but what a difficult idea it really is. Just trying to sort out its many meanings, let alone their implications, will provide us with material for many undergraduate and graduate courses, courses that could tell us as much about ourselves as a nation and a culture as they would about health.

These considerations are needed because, by the time Becker was putting together common and health, it is fairly safe to say that for many, health had become something mostly like a possession or a form of property and, thus, in our modern context, like other property, an aspect of individual identity. We tended to see health one body at a time. In both prevention and treatment, we evaluated our individual risks individually, albeit sometimes against "norms," and then we developed—or in too many cases *didn't* develop—plans for securing our health, or recovering it, individually.

It's also not just an accident that things worked out this way. The historian, Roy Porter (1997), writes:

> Western medicine...has developed radically distinctive approaches to exploring the workings of the human body in sickness and in health. These have changed the ways our culture conceives of the body and of human life. To reduce complex matters to crass terms, most peoples and most cultures the world over, throughout history, have *construed life (birth and death, sickness and health) primarily in the context of an understanding of the relations of human beings to the wider cosmos*: planets, stars, mountains, rivers, spirits and ancestors, gods and demons, the heavens and the underworld, and so forth. Some traditions, notably those reflected in Chinese and Indian learned medicine, while being concerned with the architecture of the cosmos, do not pay great attention to the supernatural. Modern western thinking, however, has become indifferent to all such elements. The West *has evolved a cul-*

ture preoccupied with the self, with the individual and his or her identity, and this quest has come to be equated with (or reduced to) the individual body and *the embodied personality,* expressed through body language. Hamlet wanted this too solid flesh to melt away. That—except in the context of slimming obsessions—is the last thing most westerners want to happen to their flesh; they want it to last as long as possible. [Emphasis added.]

This Western approach isn't entirely wrongheaded, far from it. I am reminded of Eubie Blake's answer, when in his 90s he was asked his secret for longevity and he responded: "If I'd known I was going to live this long, I would have taken better care of myself." Blake was right: For many of the leading causes of death there are behaviors (and choices) that we can identify that will either increase the chances of illness, injury, and premature death or decrease them. It seems prudent and sensible, therefore, to concentrate some of our effort at learning these things and learning how to act upon them.

The approach, however, is incomplete in several ways (as Blake's gentle irony also makes clear). The self-centered approach tends to obscure forces and conditions beyond an individual's control. It neglects context. And, as far as common health is concerned, individual risk assessments can provide opportunities to disconnect from problems and issues that aren't immediately "one's own."

We can hear this incompleteness in our national discussions of health and medicine. We experience this inadequacy on campus. Increasingly, we suffer the consequences of behavior by people who would be considered healthy individually perhaps, but whose actions undermine the academic mission, damage relationships on and off campus, and occasionally result in severe injury or accidental death. Students who could or even did pass "rigorous" physicals—many of whom are also engaged in elaborate personal fitness regimes—die of alcohol poisoning or its associated consequences, victimize others intentionally, and engage in behaviors that expose them and others to acute risks or chronic disability. Is this health?

Thinking about our common health is a way of addressing the "disequilibrium" that attaches to approaches to prevention and health that are thoroughly atomized, too dependent on individual heroic acts of rebellion from the dominant social norms, or blind to forces larger than even the most fully actualized individual. How would adding "common" to health help?

It seems to me to be an essential part of the democratic project. In examining how and when we might apply "common" to health, I think we can recover parts of our history, just as we can envision our future. Moreover, we can also examine the present, including the present state of our civic relations within a liberal democracy. Such examination is part of the process of democracy, now and always. In thinking about "common," I can hear both the echoes of our founding fathers' actions—the pledging of their lives, their fortunes, and their honor to the commonweal—and I can also glimpse the eventual fulfillment of the democratic promises they made to each other and ultimately for us and those who will follow us. The future will be marked by our discovery of the extent of our commonness with others and the implications of that commonness for our public and private lives. We hope this monograph will contribute, at least in a small way, to this exploration and that it will help in the national effort to improve education and health.

A MAP TO THIS BOOK

Each essay in this collection can stand on its own. As a collection, there is a logic to each one's inclusion and arrangement, however. Here is a map to *Learning for Our Common Health.*

In the next essay, Patsy Reed, a scientist writing while she was the chancellor of the University of North Carolina-Asheville, reflects on the role of leaders and the nature of leadership. She tells us why she regards HIV/AIDS as something that deserves and demands the attention and resources of higher education. She also claims that HIV/AIDS provides us with a set of "teachable moments" that should be seized upon, not only as part of a campus' comprehensive prevention effort, but, equally importantly, as a way of "doing" liberal education and engaging with the world beyond the campus.

The two essays that follow Dr. Reed's, both by colleagues at the University of Wisconsin, develop the two strands of our topic more comprehensively: William Cronon is Frederick Jackson Turner Professor of history, geography, and environmental studies. His essay considers the relationships between liberal learning and HIV prevention and management. He does this by enumerating and then demonstrating how the very qualities that he associates with being liberally educated are essential to really preventing HIV disease. Professor Cronon explores how understanding HIV disease depends on the illuminations and insights of many disciplines and argues that disease is always something more than a biological or virological event. Dr. Cronon says that a liberal education should be about engagement, empowerment, and community, the very qualities and conditions he suggests are necessary for overcoming disease and achieving health.

Richard Keeling is professor of medicine and director of university health services. His work on the national scene on the subject of HIV and college students is singular in its length, breadth, and effectiveness. In his essay, Dr. Keeling surveys the history of the academy's response to HIV/AIDS and finds in it valuable lessons about health and education. He shows how changes in thinking about public health—changes that he argues return public health to its roots and insist on the consideration of context and deeper, more nuanced understandings for causes of disease than the personal behaviors that expose people to harm—correspond to changes in the academy's views of learning. In the end, he shows how the very same reforms that the academy is adopting about learning are those that will improve health.

The next three essays take up specific, intentional uses of HIV/AIDS to achieve objectives that were deemed important by the leaders we surveyed: Ira Harkavy and Dan Romer, distinguished leaders in service learning from the University of Pennsylvania, outline their ideas for "strategic, academically based community scholarship and service." Recalling Dewey's "forked road situation," they see HIV/AIDS as the kind of problem that can induce learning—a learning that is designed to make a significant difference in the life conditions of those served, and not just in the students who are engaged in the service. They illustrate this idea using examples from four settings and conclude with suggestions for implementation.

Nora Kizer Bell, president of Wesleyan College, considers how the "Pandora's box" of issues raised by HIV/AIDS could be used to improve ethics courses. She shows how "respect for persons" could inform our personal behavior and how applying ethical reasoning could improve HIV/AIDS prevention and management proposals. Opposed to coercive measures alleged as necessary to achieve perfect results, Dr. Bell argues that freedom is essential to democratic, liberal learning. She concludes that a concern for freedom and for human dignity should inform our campus and broader prevention efforts.

Robert Fullilove and Mindy Thompson Fullilove, researchers in public health at Columbia University with extensive experience considering how issues of race and health intersect, provide an historical explanation for how race and racism influence health and HIV/AIDS, in particular. Arguing that any effective educational strategy has to start with understanding what people already believe, they demonstrate how an understanding of the issues of trust and truth are deeply intertwined with rumors, beliefs that all too often have some basis in fact and experience.

In the final essay, we have an account of the development of San Francisco State University's efforts regarding HIV/AIDS from its president, Robert Corrigan, and Sheila McClear, the university's director of special projects. They provide us with three snapshots of phases in this development and in so doing give us an inventory of activities and approaches that have broad application. Arguing that campus engagement with HIV transformed it for the better, they conclude by showing how campus response to HIV/AIDS actually achieved the very goals that their new campus strategic plan envisions for the whole of the university.

THE DESIGN OF OUR DESIGN

A word on the design of the book helps to recapitulate our purposes and express our hope that these essays will help leaders improve learning and health.

Our designer placed the text—with all its words, arguments, options, choices, and recommendations—against a background of blood. In doing so, he reminds us that it is, after all, in this world of blood—a world invisible to the naked eye—that HIV/AIDS plots out its cellular journey. Paul Farmer (1992), the physician and anthropologist, puts it this way:

> Although HIV is a very cosmopolitan microbe, AIDS discourse, already so abundant as to be overwhelming, has always been provincial. Were Manno or Anita or Dieudonné [three persons though whom Farmer describes HIV in Haiti] to hear the North American debates triggered by AIDS they might find them elitist struggles over goods and services long denied to the poor. Or they might deem them debates unreasonably abstract in the face of great suffering. Above all, these debates would suggest to them a vast distance, when from an intracellular parasite's point of view, the distance between us is microscopic.

In the "microscopic world," HIV encounters the drugs designed to blunt its force; here, also, it encounters the ordinary materials that will increase its potency. There is no necessary inexorability to this. Our common health depends on what we do. The splashes of blood on the bottom of the page, the blood that flows through the manuscript, and the pictures of this underworld within us—some of awesome, abstract expressionistic beauty—are meant to remind us that HIV/AIDS is ultimately anything but an abstraction.

References for this essay may be found on page 147.

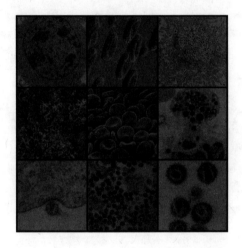

TWO

IF WE FAIL TO LEAD

Patsy B. Reed

UNIVERSITY OF NORTH CAROLINA AT ASHEVILLE

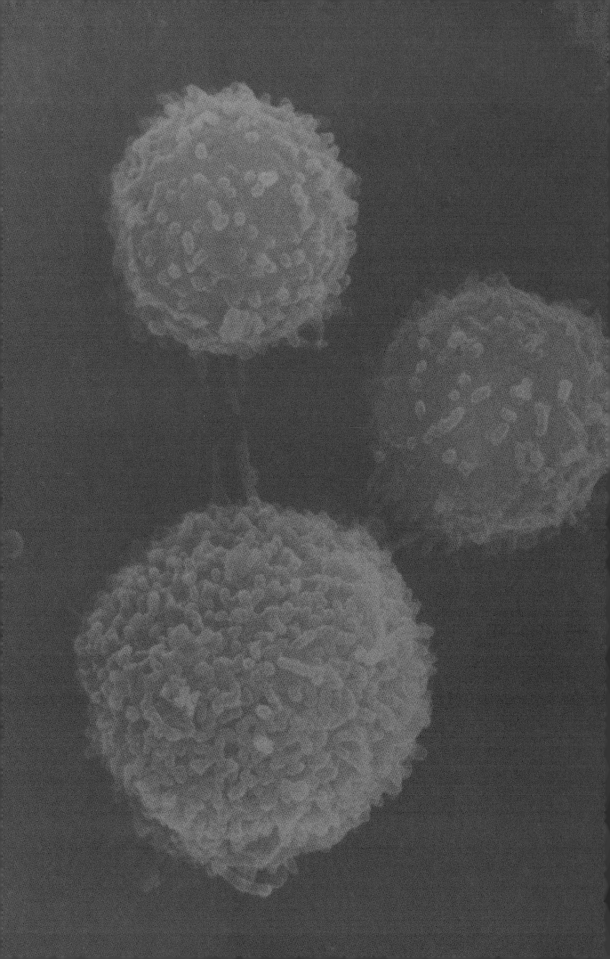

To pose the question "What will future historians say about us if we fail to lead?" might strike some as a little defensive. But asking this question helps us to think about why we should engage the many issues that HIV/AIDS throws into sharpest relief. It also suggests how we should be engaged.

There are good reasons for us to pay attention to HIV/AIDS as a disease. HIV/AIDS disproportionately affects two groups in which we have a particular interest: first, young people, and second, the families of those least-represented—whom we hope to include—in higher education; African-Americans and Latinos. Lives depend on what we do, on our campuses and in the world where we send our graduates to live and work. As our graduates begin their professional careers and make their places in their communities, what they know of health, both personal and public, and what they have learned about HIV disease and others like it will take on special significance. What they know—and how they think and act—will determine the course of their future and ours.

The complex sets of issues that HIV/AIDS embodies—indeed, health itself—are common to us all. But there is more to say. It is clear that the issues of health and disease and what to do about them will be among the most significant matters that our graduates will have to contend with in the coming century, regardless of their professional roles.

For us in higher education, HIV/AIDS then becomes two things: Fundamentally, it is a cruel disease affecting people we care about. As such, it challenges us to deploy a broad range of intellectual and other human resources to prevent and manage it. But second, HIV/AIDS is a learning opportunity—something that has provided what one might call a *national teachable moment* common to us all. It is not just one teachable moment, although HIV/AIDS has given us many specific moments that teach many specific things. HIV/AIDS provides a continuous stream of teachable moments. In the spirit of making something good happen from what is—like so many other diseases—an otherwise tragic set of circumstances, I want to suggest that there is "gift" in HIV/AIDS. This gift, if we choose to accept it, will allow us to improve our understanding and to turn that new understanding into improvements in health, in higher education, and in our communities.

TRADITIONS IN HIGHER EDUCATION

We say with justification that our nation's institutions of higher education are the envy of the world. Our quality, diversity, and record in both conserving and creating knowledge are unsurpassed. The democratic ideals that we embrace are given new life each day by the millions of students—from all parts of our society and indeed the world—whom we enroll in our many programs. Our span is vast, from the children studying in our lab schools and learning in our day care centers to the senior citizens enrolled in our elder programs. We lead the world in basic research. In an intensely practical way, we are vitally engaged in the economic welfare of our communities, regions, and nation.

We have many cherished traditions, such as academic freedom, decentralization of authority—even arguing. These are great sources of strength. In the face of a claimed crisis, these conditions also slow our capacity to organize ourselves to apply our talents and skills with any predictable efficiency. In our culture—committed as we are to deliberation, respect for differing views, and debate about basic purposes—there inheres a resistance to jumping on anybody's bandwagon. While this resistance certainly means that many bad impulses will be chilled, it can also mean that some opportunities to do good things will be missed.

Debate and disagreement about the fundamental meaning or importance of something or about choosing a course of action will bring some of these traditions to the foreground. Faced with being urged to march in a particular direction or staying clear of the complex issue, some might say that the prudent course is one of disengagement. But what if disengagement carries with it the loss of a significant opportunity to make a difference—or change the course of history? In such an event, we would surely have to face the probability that our future judges—the future historians—will accuse us of irresponsibility, cowardice, or worse.

Provocative comparisons of HIV to other plagues have been made. There are similarities. What are our obligations in a time of plague? We know more today—more that can be put in the service of fighting disease—than our forebears at the medieval universities of Paris and Bologna did during the Black Death. Would we accept idleness or half-measures from our forebears if they had given less than their full measure in the time of their plague? What would they expect from us today, in the face of what some have called our new plague? Would anything less than our best efforts be acceptable? I think not.

IMMUNITY AS METAPHOR

One particular biological aspect of HIV is that it somehow affects the body's immune response. It forces those who have it to face invasions in their lives that would otherwise have gone unnoticed. Insults that ordinarily would have little chance of succeeding against the body's defenses suddenly (or gradually, as the case may be) take on new powers, new ferocity, new saliency. Let's hold this idea in our minds as a metaphor, for a moment.

When I think about most learning, I find myself thinking about how much of it is methodical, cumulative, leveraged on what has been learned, on principles already mastered and skills acquired. There is a quietness—a latency—in all this. Much of what we have to learn, we have to learn this way. But I am also impressed by the kind of learning that comes—indeed, sometimes explodes—from the teachable moment: the kind of event that eats at and tests our defenses, invades our security, afflicts our comfort. Like the opportunistic infection, this learning allows something to take on a new meaning, a new power that it didn't previously have, a chance to make a connection not made so far. Learning becomes an experience that generates a reaction, stimulates and challenges defenses, opens new pathways, and leaves the learner changed in some significant way.

This is precisely the result we desire when we seek to immunize someone: to stimulate a set of mechanisms, a struggle, and, by so doing, to strengthen the organism and its possibility of resisting damage. On a biological level, this is what we hope will happen for HIV, as well. But I am speaking metaphorically about the social body's reaction to it.

We can say that on campus our defenses, i.e., our immunity, seemed sufficient at first. AIDS was not "our" disease or "our" problem. It was scary, but ignorable. We fought it off without knowing we were even fighting it. Then a new mutation occurred. AIDS became a disease of a few of us. In many instances, we conspired in silence to keep it that way. Then, in another mutation, AIDS turned into something that could affect all of us. But the chances of that happening for any one of us seemed so remote that it was as if the whole force of the disease was somehow remote. We inoculated ourselves with a little AIDS so that most of us could become immune to a lot of it. Now we could feel a little better about ourselves. We could go on to other things.

In the midst of all this, however, several things seemed to be happening in the real, biological and political world of AIDS: the infection continued to grow among the young, the conditions around the world worsened, and advances in treatment resulted in longer lives and more expensive treatment, but accentuated greater disparities in access to care. And now this disease—and our efforts to manage it morally, politically, and medically—gives us the hardest, most vexing, and apparently intractable questions imaginable. Some are not new: They are enduring, ancient questions. Others are more distinctly modern, by-products of our development and progress. Let me suggest just a few:

- What is the relationship of knowledge to action, or how does what we know affect what we do?

- What is our responsibility to those beyond our political borders whose health and welfare are intimately linked to what we do, or to those within our borders?

- Now that we know how to extend life, on what grounds will we allocate the resources (or the drugs, therapies, treatments) to grant extensions to some and not to others?

- In our personal relationships, what do we owe one another—how much regard and how much honesty, about ourselves, our intentions, our desires?

Beyond these questions, HIV/AIDS leaves us with other legacies of a more personal and moral nature: lessons to be learned in human dignity, respect for others, the duty to protect others, struggles over and obligations to self-discipline and restraint. It both quickens and challenges our spirituality. It acquaints us with grief—the loss of our sons and daughters, our loved ones, our colleagues and friends.

In getting to know HIV/AIDS we may have also been given a glimpse of the future. Perhaps HIV/AIDS is not some isolated aberration that will go away as some other lost disease, like smallpox. Rather, HIV/AIDS may be a kind of disease that will be very much with us in the future: diseases of new encounters, diseases of changing and mutating organisms that evade treatment and control. If this view is correct, then the late twentieth and early twenty-first centuries may be consumed by attention to new viral illnesses that challenge the body's immune defenses. This will be our future. If this is true, then what we learn about and from HIV/AIDS will have utility and value well beyond the specifics of HIV/AIDS itself.

But, after all, who can predict the future? Let's say HIV/AIDS is a unique phenomenon and that it is on the verge of becoming a "been there" issue. We are still left with a whole set of issues—many public policy matters that will have deep effects in each of our lives—that involve health and that will take on growing significance in the next century.

POLICY CONSIDERATIONS

Let me suggest just a few questions within a broad range of public policy considerations that are post-modern. Indeed, as we saw before, some are the by-products of the advances we have made:

- What are we to do about the growing gap between the medical "haves" and "have-nots," here and abroad? The emergence of new drug therapies gives a new, literal meaning to the question of who will live and who will die.

- How will we balance the costs/expenses for the acute care needs of older Americans or persons with diseases and disabilities with the more elusive but compelling prevention needs of younger people?

- How will we pay for anything other than the costs associated with the retirements and health of the baby boomer generation?

- Should "who you are" determine what you get? Does our sense of the status of a "victim" determine the urgency and comprehensiveness of our response to that person's needs? Should it? Relatedly, if I could prevent harm from coming to me and I do not act to prevent it, should I forfeit my claim to support for subsequent needs?

- How do we balance our sense of the prudential or practical solutions to something with our principled concerns about or objections to something?

- How do we contend with theories of disease that are deeply intertwined with distrust for authorities within the dominant culture? The conspiracy theories that abound about HIV/AIDS might seem preposterous to some of us, but they are credible to others whose ancestors were the objects of medical experimentation.

- How can our system of health care—one that is so brilliantly capable of rendering heroic care for acute conditions—be re-engineered to provide equally good management for chronic conditions?

In our democracy, we should resist a temptation to regard these and like questions as technical matters reserved for experts: They affect us all. They shape important personal questions: freedom and self-determination, opportunities for equal protection, chances to realize our personal aspirations and our futures.

And so, keeping in mind our mission as colleges, we might ask: Are our graduates prepared to engage in the discussions, advance the knowledge, and find the solutions to these new dilemmas? Are they as good as they can be at the hard work of translating what they know into effective strategies to protect themselves and others?

HEALTH AND EDUCATION

Health is a matter of great common concern—something that is both personal/private but also something that we all share, in our families, and more broadly, with others in our communities, and indeed, with people we will never meet. Health is also a good candidate for an organizing idea—a thematic focus—for parts of an undergraduate education. Of course, there are other useful organizing ideas: the environment, international peace, social justice, the meanings of nationhood and national identity, internationalism, and so on. A case can be made for each of these and others—and fortunately we do not have to choose just one.

What choosing an organizing idea does, though, is to provide a good strategy for teaching and learning. Professor June Osborn, former chair of the President's National Commission on AIDS, once called AIDS "multidisciplinary trouble." By so doing she suggests that we will require the resources, insights, and traditions of a variety of disciplines to grasp its many meanings.

I find HIV/AIDS so compelling not only because it is a matter of life and death. May I suggest that HIV/AIDS is almost unique in that it sits at the intersection of so much that is happening in the lives of our students. It is a problem that can be prevented by education and that will be ameliorated by people who are effectively educated. Ultimately HIV/AIDS may be eliminated through advances we make in education. Education, it can be argued, can be the whole answer in HIV prevention—though resources, funds, good policies, and services are surely needed to help the more than one in 250 Americans who are currently HIV-positive, not to mention the millions of people around the world who lack access to effective medical services.

What kind of education? It is in thinking about this question that we also begin to think about how to improve education. There is a reciprocal relationship here: how we can improve public health by improving education, and how we can improve education by focusing on health.

The approach I am advocating will require us to confront gaps in our current knowledge and understanding of virology and immunology, certainly, but of human behavior, as well. It will require interdisciplinarity and collaboration across disciplines, between academic and student life functions. It points up the need for community involvement and service. It demands that we think beyond the campus, beyond our towns, and beyond our borders. It forces us to confront significant cultural and political conflicts. This approach insists on connecting theory and practice. It generates controversy, stirs emotions and passions, leaves us bewildered, challenged, and sometimes hopeful, and it will lead to new understanding. But isn't that what a good education is all about?

I believe that we need to think about and come to better understand HIV/AIDS and health. The lessons—the gifts, as I have said—HIV/AIDS has to teach us are volatile mixtures. Handling these materials will require our thoughtfulness, wit, ingenuity, sensitivity, and creativity. It will require courage, patience, and respect for the power—and sometimes for the fragility—of the many elements and forces in the reactions. But I would say that this is our reason for being. This is our mission.

LEADING ON CAMPUS

So what about leading? How do we get where we want to be? Well, thinking is a good place to begin, as always. And listening is helpful too. Reflecting on my own experience at Asheville, I have been encouraged by the reaction of our campus and community to our theater department's recent set of performances of the play "Angels in America." And beyond my own campus, I was heartened to learn that more than 70 percent of my fellow presidents and chancellors who responded to the AAC&U survey thought that it was very important or essential that students learn about HIV/AIDS in their coursework.

We are interested, many of us, in how we can combine the efforts of our academic and student life offerings to the benefit of students. And though we should be conscious of what one of my fellow presidents called "our natural cognitive bias," I do think we need to explore how collaborations and the intellectualizing or problematizing of the issues of health can help support specific changes in behavior. By making these issues matters for academic inquiry, we may improve the effectiveness of our curricular efforts to promote health.

Before concluding, let me offer a few words about leadership. The best leadership is the leadership of and by example. I'll sketch out two things: first, what leaders can and should do. Second, what leaders need to help them lead. These are simple ideas, but often not simple things.

What leaders can do:

- We can help create a climate that encourages taking on hard topics. We can do this by example, and we can show respect and give encouragement to those who do. If I contributed to the success of "Angels in America" on my campus, it was simply in setting a tone that encourages exploration of difficult issues.

- We can help prepare those who are legally responsible for the work that we do for the possible controversy and difficulty that taking on hard issues may generate. We can "manage controversy"—sometimes. I think of our obligation to communicate with our boards of trustees, our alumni, our local community organizations, and to be attentive to their concerns.

- We can commit resources, including our own time and effort, to help make things happen. I want to quickly add that one very appealing dimension of using health and HIV/AIDS as an organizing theme and topic in courses is that we already have resources committed to this learning. The direction I am suggesting asks us to re-think not what we are doing, but how we are doing it. We may need to add support for development, etc., but the talent—both faculty and student—is already present on our campuses.

• We can "stick around for the answer." I am reminded of Bacon's essay "Of truth" where he writes, "What is truth? said jesting Pilate; and would not stay for an answer." Leaders need to stay for an answer. We need to persist, not just launch things and walk away when things get troublesome, as they sometimes do.

And what do leaders need?

• We need intellectual rigor (not rigidity) and honesty, from those who engage in this and all work, along with a commitment to examine and evaluate efforts undertaken.

• We need advice and help, the benefit of a broad range of human experience and knowledge, and a sensitivity to differences in beliefs and values.

• We need creativity—a willingness to try new things, to try things in new ways.

• We need collaboration that focuses on results—and not simply the discovery of mutual interests and opportunities.

In the end, we have much to give one another and much to gain from one another. Good results will happen with greater certainty if we use our imaginations, occasionally suspend our disbelief, and persistently think about the larger goals we all share. Sacrifices may be entailed and much of what we need to do will be hard work. But I am left with the sense that it is to hard tasks that we must commit ourselves. It is to leading on matters that require leadership that we must focus our energies. Presidents set the tone and lead by creating a climate that encourages thought and dialogue.

I serve on a leadership advisory board for AAC&U's Program for Health and Higher Education. Also on that board is the president of San Francisco State University, the leader of an urban university literally at the epicenter of the AIDS epidemic, the original ground zero in the U.S., you might say. Dr. Corrigan says that no part of SFSU is not infiltrated—forever changed—by the emotional, physical, intellectual, and cultural presence of HIV disease. The student newspaper carries a weekly AIDS obituary column. On a day-in, day-out basis, the students, faculty, and staff live with an acute sense of loss.

Another board member is Thomas Hearn, the president of Wake Forest University. Winston-Salem is no epicenter of the epidemic, but it is a major intellectual center. And, unlike public San Francisco State, Wake Forest is a private university, one that is historically affiliated with the Baptist church. Partly inspired by the death of a beloved friend, President Hearn, a philosopher by training, has taken it upon himself to talk about HIV/AIDS to all Wake Forest first-year students. He thinks that students need to think about important and big things, and he hopes to help them in that thinking—and, perhaps, to influence them to take care of themselves and others. His taking this on represents his own contribution, his own teaching by example, his own sense of his duty to students.

I come from the sublimely beautiful place of Asheville—surrounded by mountains, remote in many ways, but like much of North Carolina, occupying a place somewhere between sylvan isolation and a growing cosmopolitan, commercial, and cultural engagement with peoples around the world. It is tempting—gazing at the mountains that give us our motto and our inspiration—and it might even be safe to feel immune from many things: from forces, events, and perils raging outside what seems to be our remote part of the world.

But I have a conviction that there is a connection between what we do at North Carolina's public liberal arts university and what happens in our city, our region, the nation, and the world. Our students deserve not only the comforts of isolation; they require the challenges of engagements with the greatest issues we face now and in the future. So I come to this work because I want to see how—by respecting our traditions and drawing on our strengths—we can seize on the teachable national moment, the common event of HIV/AIDS.

The teachable moment is given to us to make a difference for our students' health and education.

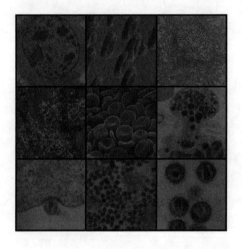

THREE

HIV, Health, and Liberal Education

William J. Cronon
University of Wisconsin

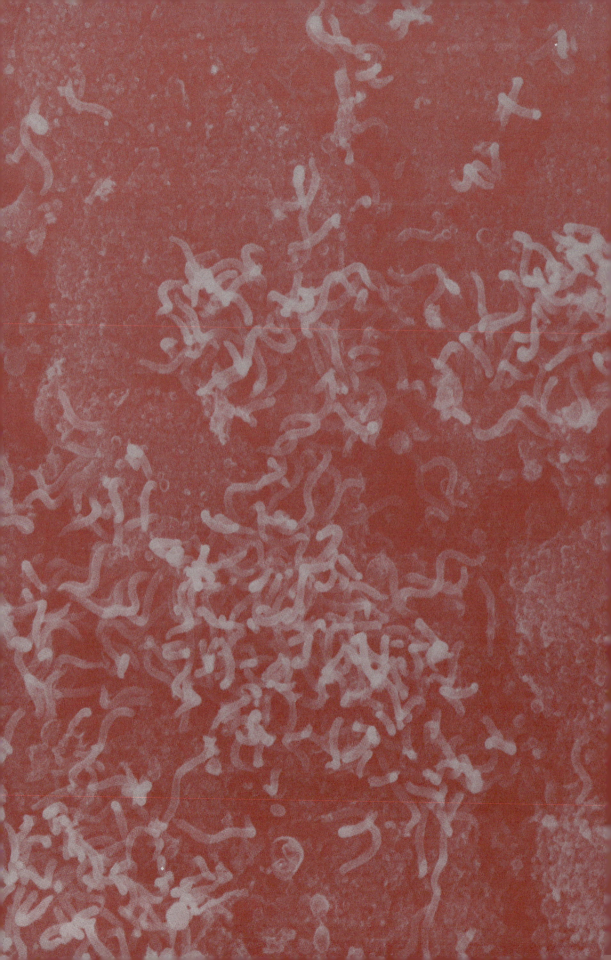

The audience for the speech from which this essay was adapted had been warned that several speakers who had no specific credentials to do so were going to stand in front of them to hold forth on the subject of HIV/AIDS. I felt like a prize trophy in this effort: I arrived at the meeting with the sense that I was less qualified to speak on HIV/AIDS and health education in the modern college and university than any other single person in the room.

I have little specific background in the study of HIV/AIDS except in my identity as an environmental historian: a historian who looks at changing interactions between people in the natural world (which inevitably include disease).On the brighter side, in the last couple of years I have been devoting much of my time to trying to figure out how we can do a better job of teaching undergraduates.

These interests have led me to think a lot about what it means to be a liberally educated person. But as I thought about it, it became clear to me that I couldn't give a speech on what it means to be a liberally educated person unless I could somehow persuade the audience that liberal education was somehow relevant to HIV/AIDS. I had been asked to grapple with questions about the relationship of education and health and HIV/AIDS, and that is my aim in this essay.

To do this, I will have to spend a fair amount of time trying to link my vision of undergraduate education with the many issues raised by HIV/AIDS and disease prevention in general. I have to confess that I struggled a bit with the aims of those who want us to focus on these things: Is the goal to promote HIV/AIDS education as an end in itself, or is the goal to promote HIV/AIDS education as a means to the larger end of promoting a better, more integrated sense of health education in undergraduate and other forms of teaching? And still more broadly, what is the relationship of HIV/AIDS to my own goal of improving undergraduate education in general? How are these things knit together? How generalizable are the insights that come from thinking about these things? How broadly can they extend? How many people, how many subjects, how many parts and practices in our lives can they touch?

My own belief is that we should think very broadly indeed about the ways in which a focus on HIV/AIDS can arc out into the larger world of the academy. Toward that end, I want to offer some meditations on education generally, reflect upon the phenomenon of HIV/AIDS, and end with some thoughts on what it means to be a liberally educated person.

This essay is adapted from remarks made by the author at the Leadership Conference sponsored by AAC&U, NAFEO, and NASPA in Madison, WI on April 2-4, 1998. The final section is drawn, with permission, from his article, "Only Connect," published in the Fall 1998 issue of *The American Scholar*.

THE PARADOX OF SPECIALIZATION

I have recently been involved in a number of reforms at UW-Madison directed toward improving undergraduate education, all gathered under the heading "The Pathways to Excellence Project." These reforms have included things like a new research program that tries to get freshmen and sophomores into research laboratories and into archives working directly as research assistants for faculty members and a new writing fellows program that has undergraduates serving as co-teachers with faculty members in trying to improve the writing skills of other students. Most dramatically—and most consuming of my life—has been a new living-learning community on our campus, Chadbourne Residential College, opened in August 1997. Students, faculty members, and staff from student affairs, health services, and health education have all been intimately involved in this residential college project. One of our goals is to try to figure out what it means to nurture a real community among undergraduates who often experience these enormous state research universities as very alienating, very massive and anonymous institutions, the very antithesis of community. By community, I mean a gathering of human beings that has face-to-face relations at its center, a gathering of human beings who, ideally at least, actually know each other's names.

What's important about these several initiatives is that they share certain common themes: They are not essentially curricular, none of them is required, and none of them is something we demand or expect of all undergraduates coming through our university. Rather, they are "pathways to excellence." Here, excellence is designed and defined as a pathway that students choose for themselves not because of grades or credits, but because of an inner passion they have discovered in themselves. This passion marks the way toward a life journey. Students are no longer going to school because someone has told them what they must do to fulfill requirements. Rather, they've chosen where they're going for themselves—they have a direction that is their own.

None of these new initiatives are honors programs, although honor students often benefit from them. The programs are not limited to a small, elite group of students defined by anything so narrow as a grade point average. Rather, they are for students who are actively engaged with their own educations.

Our goals for the Pathways to Excellence Project programs are very simple. I hope they are also the goals we all try to keep at the center of our educational efforts. Very abstractly put, they are about engagement, empowerment, and community. Such goals of course mean nothing until they become a lived reality. But I would argue that, at this abstract level, these core values—engagement, empowerment, and community—should be the goals of any educational institution that hopes to prepare its students for a life of citizenship, meaning a life that contributes to the communities of which they are a part.

Yet I would argue that all too often colleges and universities are not about these things. Rather, they are about disengagement, disempowerment, and an experience of mass culture and mass bureaucratic interaction that is the furthest thing from what we would want a real community to be.

Why is that? Why do we organize these institutions in such a way that we don't consistently deliver to our students engagement, empowerment, and community? There are lots of reasons. One that I want to concentrate on here, because I think it relates to the issue of health and HIV/AIDS, can be seen as a paradox arising from specialization. It flows from one of the great virtues especially of the research universities, and in fact characterizes all institutions of higher learning. It is a virtue that all too easily becomes a vice.

For the most part, university and college teaching is done by people who are trained in what we call "the disciplines," people who have become experts in a particular body of specialized knowledge. This specialized knowledge is what they seek to impart to their students. It's not an accident that we do this. There are very important reasons why sharing the disciplines with the next generation is a chief task of colleges and universities.

The power of disciplinary specialization arises from the insights that come from viewing the world through a very particular lens. The rigor comes from viewing the world through blinders. Economists know rigor because of the tightly focused way economics defines human behavior and directs attention to a useful fiction called "the market." Epidemiologists understand disease via a narrow but powerful set of tools that allow them to test assumptions about the ways certain organisms move through human communities. These narrow disciplinary perspectives are not to be belittled. The rigor that would be impossible without the disciplines is crucial to any vision of learning in the modern world. The expertise that the disciplines make possible is fundamentally about gaining the power to act and make a difference in the world. I say power because we know that disciplinary knowledge enables us to interact with the phenomena that we are trying to change in ways we know will be effective.

Surely any student moving through our campuses should aspire to attain the benefits of the disciplines—the insights, the rigor, the power, and the expertise that are the gifts that the disciplines hold out to us. But just as surely we must all recognize—at least those of us who are committed to undergraduate teaching as opposed to graduate training—that disciplinary specialization and rigor are not by themselves enough.

The narrow perspective that comes from focusing on a small domain brings great power but also obscures from view much of the world. The power is bought with the same act of focusing that obscures the rest of the world. As a result, we're all too apt—because of our disciplinary power and specialization and expertise—to miss, to render invisible, to erase the interconnections and synergies that have been defined out of existence by the blinders we've chosen to put on.

It is not an accident that we have chosen to erase these interconnections. That is why, when we talk in an idealized way about the goals of undergraduate education, we rarely say that disciplinary specialization is what we're mainly after. We reserve such specialization for post-baccalaureate training. We imagine that the graduate schools, the law schools, the business schools, and the medical schools are where true professional specialization, true disciplined knowledge, happens. We say that what we want for undergraduates is a broader, more liberal sense of what education means.

INTERDISCIPLINARY BRIDGES TO LIBERAL LEARNING

When I use the words liberal education, as I'll do repeatedly here, I'll use "liberal" in the original etymological sense of the word: education for human freedom, education for the fulfillment of human talent and human promise. Liberal education aspires to take the raw material that each of us has within ourselves and liberates that potential, that talent, so we can act as free agents in the world. As part of this process, we come to recognize that the world constrains us, disciplines us, in many different ways. But we also learn to navigate these constraints and disciplines in ways that render us effective. The liberal part of liberal education asks students to become educated to see the world whole, expansively, inclusively, with an eye toward the freedom that comes from a liberal learning that refuses to be blinded by disciplinary walls.

I would be disingenuous if I denied to you my own sense that we're not very good at this. We do a poor job in general of modeling this sense of interconnectedness as teachers. We say the words, but we don't enact them. Academic specialists all too often teach their specialties even when they are addressing first-year students. They do this without ever stopping to ask what those specialties are contributing, not to disciplinary knowledge, but to liberal learning, learning for freedom, learning for human growth. An economist teaches Economics 101 because she imagines that economics is somehow important. A historian teaches American history because he imagines that American history is somehow important. The same goes for biology or chemistry or whatever the subject may be. The subject gets taught as if it were an end in and of itself, something essential for students to know. And this seems to me a serious error in the way we conceive of the goals of undergraduate education.

The way I would put it, as I think about what we offer students with our disciplinary knowledge, is that we teachers—in our passion for our particular, peculiar, individual subjects—are a bridge for the journey those students are on, but we ourselves don't know the end of their journey. We do know that it is almost never the place where we ourselves ended up. They are headed somewhere else.

If our disciplines are to serve the larger goal of liberal learning, we must recognize that we are a bridge for a journey whose end we do not know and that we ourselves will never see. We must therefore think about the kind of bridge we want to be: How capaciously and generously do we want our teaching to serve as a pathway our students will travel toward destinations different from our own? Unless we ask this question in all seriousness, our disciplines are not likely to contribute very much to liberal learning, learning for human freedom. Yet too often we ignore this question and pretend that it doesn't matter. Economics or history or chemistry—these are the sum total of what we seek to teach.

Unfortunately, I would say that this is often just as true of those of us who are committed to interdisciplinary knowledge. Whether we require of students a core curriculum or environmental literacy or even knowledge about health or HIV/AIDS, if we conceive of such requirements in too narrowly focused or disciplined a way, we are likely to fall into the same trap of imagining that the means to the end—the bridge we are serving for our students' journey, the bridge whose end we do not yet know—is the end itself.

These subjects that we are trying to share with our students—environmental literacy or HIV/AIDS—are they a means to the end of liberal, engaged, empowered, community-minded people, or are they ends in themselves? The answer must clearly be that they are both. We want our students to come out of our teaching with a sense of liberal learning on the one hand, and we also want them to know something about HIV/AIDS or environmental problems or whatever it is we want them to know about the world. But if I had to choose between these aims, I'd pick liberal learning rather than any particular concrete object of liberal learning that I happen bring into the classroom as my particular passion. And however strongly we feel about the importance of HIV/AIDS education, my goal here is to try to persuade us to do the same.

One reason is that it's always good to remember the resistance in students that comes from being told they must learn something. It's also good to remember the passion that comes from knowledge that we've discovered on our own. Remember the old saw about "leading a horse to water but not forcing that horse to drink." But also recall the miracle that we all witness from time to time in our classrooms when lightning strikes. A student encounters a subject, a light suddenly shines, that student falls in love with learning—and we can never explain why it happened to that particular student on that particular day in that particular way. This is the miracle of a student and a teacher connecting with each other in ways one could never have predicted. We could not have known that that particular relationship was going to yield that particular set of insights. Knowing this, we need to recognize that different classrooms will offer different forms of lightning for different students. Accepting the uncertainty and unpredictability of such miracles is a condition of teaching. So just as I'm disinclined to require that students take mandatory courses in a particular kind of history, so too am I disinclined to require environmental literacy, or, for that matter, to require knowledge of HIV/AIDS.

Let me restate this in a more affirmative way. I think we are more likely to attain our goal of helping students understand and engage issues like HIV/AIDS if they encounter this subject as a means to their own ends, as a vehicle for their own learning, rather than as a vehicle for our proselytizing them about our ends, our convictions about what we think they should know.

The Cultural Construction of Disease

I can illustrate what I am saying here with a couple of stories that come out of my own disciplinary blinders and lenses. I am an environmental historian. I look at the history of people's interactions with the natural world. Therefore, my core subject inevitably has a lot to do with epidemic disease. We can't talk about people's interactions with the natural world without thinking a lot about the environment which is our own bodies and the ways our bodies relate to the other environment which is the world beyond the boundaries our own bodies' walls. I am thus biased to see HIV disease as part of a centuries-old process involving the migration of infectious disease historically linked to the worldwide expansion of European empires over the past 500 years. I see HIV/AIDS through my disciplinary lenses as an environmental historian.

Probably the most dramatic episode that I teach in my classes and that I've written about in my own books is the infection, through "virgin soil epidemics" as they're sometimes called, of Native American peoples in the western hemisphere following the arrival of European, Asian, and African peoples traveling across the Atlantic and Pacific oceans. The story involves the introduction of very old-fashioned kinds of organisms like measles or smallpox into a human population that essentially had no immunological history with those organisms. Massive mortalities ensued, with death rates sometimes on the order of 50-90 percent in the course of just a few days or weeks. The associated depopulation of the American landscape flowing from the epidemics had a host of cultural consequences. We can see the cascade of effects this implied for the American landscape in the cultural meanings that native peoples and Europeans attached to these diseases: as God's justification, God's clearing of the New England landscape for the invading colonists, removing the Indians to make it possible for colonists to settle. My main point here relating to HIV/AIDS is that HIV/AIDS is an older story than it appears to be on the surface. There are many, many historical analogs to HIV/AIDS, even though it of course has its own peculiar horrors. These are not quite like the horrors of smallpox as suffered by Aztec or other Indians in the New World. But their stories at least suggest questions we should ask about the subtle cultural complexities that inhere in an epidemic like HIV/AIDS.

I say this because unless we understand diseases are not just biological phenomena but also cultural phenomena, we are likely to misunderstand the nature of what we are looking at when we study it. To make this point more forcefully I want to move to a more modern epidemic and a wonderful book written in 1962 by Charles Rosenberg, *The Cholera Years*. In it, he narrates three cholera epidemics that occurred during the nineteenth century, one in 1832, one in 1849, and one in 1866. He uses these three epidemics as evidence that cholera in 1849 didn't look quite as it did in 1832, and it looked still more different in 1866. He argues that it was, in effect, a different disease, even though the same infectious agent may have been tied to the different cultural forms the disease took. Essentially, he uses the contrast of the 1832 and 1866 epidemics to say that Americans and Europeans during this period moved away from a view of disease in which the principal causes of cholera were miasma (bad air, bad atmosphere) and the susceptibility of immoral people to cholera infection. Miasma and immorality explained cholera in 1832. By 1866, the arrival of a revolutionary new germ theory of disease had utterly changed the way people conceived of the infection and the way it moved through human populations. So, if you want to read this story in a particular way, it becomes one of the great heroic narratives of nineteenth-century medicine. All of a sudden, we have powerful new tools which mean that the 1866 cholera epidemic will be the last meaningful occurrence of cholera in the United States for at least the next 130 years. Now the quarantine of infected patients, the burning of their clothes, the cleaning of their houses by the Board of Health, but most especially the discovery of the linkage of cholera to the water supply, coupled with the advent and proliferation of sewage systems and public water sources: all of these interventions represent a triumph of modern medicine and the control of cholera as an infectious disease.

But here, too, there are subtle lessons relative to my earlier point about disciplinary knowledge. If we interpret the lesson of those epidemics and of Rosenberg's book *The Cholera Years* too narrowly, as Rosenberg himself does not, we will miss all sorts of important contexts. His most important point concerns the cultural construction of disease. Cholera in 1832 is different from cholera in 1866 in a deeply non-trivial way.

The fact that people experienced these "choleras" differently, that they behaved toward them in radically different ways, made cholera literally a different illness, a different disease. The set of transformations that cholera underwent over the course of the nineteenth century are deeply analogous to the phenomena we are living through as we grapple with the HIV/AIDS epidemic. HIV, both as an organism and as a human idea, is undergoing the same kind of complicated cultural evolution as cholera as we struggle to understand not just the biology but everything else associated with the disease.

Here's the take-home lesson from *The Cholera Years* that will finally carry me more directly to HIV/AIDS. The germ theory is something that we classically celebrate as the heroic insight of nineteenth century medicine. It is the triumph that moved us toward modern medicine in ways human beings had never understood before. That triumph of nineteenth-century medicine is of course the foundation for medicine as we practice it today. But this very triumph tempts us toward an associated vice, which involves over-emphasizing one particular causal theory of disease. The virtue of the germ theory was to give us a causal agent for disease. The vice of the germ theory was to construct that agent too narrowly, so that the organism itself became the disease, thereby obscuring all the associated elements that conspire together to define the lived reality and meaning of that disease for the human beings it affects. Thus, the very power of the germ theory that is its greatest virtue also tempts us to see "the germ" as the sole cause of an illness. This vision of a sole effective cause became the foundation of the discipline called medicine, a discipline which sees the treatment of the infected organism as the essential disciplinary problem and sees as its own disciplinary agenda the proper treatment of the infected organism—as opposed to imagining different definitions of what might constitute health, or imagining different ways of defining the nature of illness.

Here, of course, we can make a pretty obvious connection to HIV/AIDS. If HIV is the infectious agent, then AIDS is the disease, and they are not at all the same thing. Like any other infectious agent, HIV, when viewed through the lens of Charles Rosenberg's *The Cholera Years*, can remind us that no virus or bacteria can stand all by itself as an adequate explanation for why people fall sick and sometimes die. Explaining the nature of disease is much less simple than merely pointing to a particular organism that happens to invade a particular body. The infectious agent is only the beginning of the story—though, Lord knows, it's a complicated enough beginning. Trying to figure out the biology and chemistry of the protein design of a particular virus and the ways it organizes and interacts with the cells it invades is a crucial task. I hope no one concludes from what I'm saying here about the cultural construction of disease that

I'm belittling the insights that flow from biological perspectives on what HIV is all about and how the disease operates as it does. Biological perspectives are crucial. But there are lots and lots of other questions about HIV that are just as important. There are, for instance, questions about geographic location, how the organism is distributed, how the people it infects are distributed through space, and how that space reflects in turn questions of international boundaries, social class, ethnic and racial identity, constructions of gender, behavioral characteristics, and so on. Each of these has a peculiar geography of its own, a geography that is linked to the transmission of the organism and the manifestations of the disease.

PATTERNS OF HIV ON A BROAD CONTEMPORARY FRAMEWORK

Now, there are many other cultural constructions of the phenomenon called HIV or AIDS. What I'll do here, quickly, is just gesture at the many elements that come together to form this great kaleidoscope called HIV. These will suggest how the state of our particular medical theories at a given moment—like the medical theories associated with miasma and then with germs in 1832 and 1866 for the disease called cholera—lead us to tell stories in certain ways and not others about the cause, treatment, and outcome of the disease. The ways we tell these stories often shape what we will and will not allow ourselves to see during the course of the infection. Stories have enormous power to affect what we are willing to include within the frame of what does and does not count as the disease, what we will and will not consider as relevant in the people who are living through it. Here are some questions that we might consider: What is the culture of medical expertise? Who controls knowledge? What is the guild that possesses information defining the disease? How does this expertise shape treatment? How do protocols for new medical testing determine access to treatments? In the course of double blind experiments, do certain people and not others get access to treatment? Are some experiments exported to certain groups of people and not others, and if so, how do these groups reflect the racial and class politics associated with such investigations? How does the cost of producing, distributing, and marketing new therapies, particularly drug treatments, reflect the political economy of the corporations which deliver these therapies to the marketplace? How do systems of delivery determine who will and will not have access to therapies? How do international conditions govern the movement of disease across international boundaries? As was the case with of miasma and cholera, how do cultural assumptions and moralizing attitudes govern the ways infected individuals are perceived, both by others and by themselves? How do responses to an infectious agent interact with cultural definitions of personal and political liberty? What's the linkage of the virus to democracy or personal freedom? How do people who are differently positioned in society perceive their own vulnerability to the possibility of infection? And how—in the act of perceiving themselves as vulnerable or not vulnerable—do they separate themselves from the people that they perceive as being more vulnerable than themselves? How does this sense of separation articulate class, gender, and other kinds of boundaries within the culture? How do these boundaries affect perceptions of who is regarded as susceptible, or weak, or punishable relative to the supposed "vice" that the disease represents? How do the miasma controversies of the 1832 cholera epidemic get recapitulated in the HIV/AIDS epidemic?

My point in all of this, to go back to what I said earlier about the germ theory, is that our disciplinary knowledge—whatever our perspective and whatever our discipline might be—tempts us to see mainly the proximate causes that our discipline teaches us to see in the phenomenon we're trying to explain. We see the most immediate cause—HIV—but not a host of ancillary causes, the necessary but not sufficient causes, the contributing and ancillary causes, that come together to reproduce the phenomenon.

The other moral I would draw from the HIV/AIDS story, a moral I find extraordinarily heartening and one of the most amazing features of this particular epidemic, brings me back to my earlier theme of undergraduate education. The HIV/AIDS story teaches that an engaged, empowered, community-minded group of people—including patients, their partners, their friends, their families, and the health professionals associated with them—can basically seize control of their own illness, wrest knowledge of the disease from all sorts of hierarchies that are not eager to give up control of that knowledge, and force a whole series of complicated changes in the culture. AIDS has been a struggle over who does and does not have access to knowledge, who does and does not participate in the cultural construction of the disease. Who has the right to interpret the meaning of a disease and determine the way that it's treated? The moral of the AIDS epidemic is that the answers to these questions should include many more people than just medical experts, and that is a net gain for us all.

HIV/AIDS AS OPPORTUNITY FOR ENGAGING WITH THE COMMUNITY

I have described all this very abstractly indeed. My hope is that anyone reading this will have real flesh-and-blood human beings leap to mind as vivid examples of the phenomena I have described so academically, so bloodlessly. Abstract, academic phenomena like these always manifest themselves, make themselves real, in real human lives. One of the most important tasks of education, to go back to my earlier theme of teaching, is to make the word real, to find flesh and blood in the abstractions that our disciplines encourage us to see (and not see) out there in the world.

For me, each of the general phenomena concerning HIV which I have mentioned is also an educational hook. It is a connection, a way of linking AIDS to a larger set of educational agendas that are medical but also philosophical, historical, sociological, economic, international, political, and many other things. This means that the struggle against HIV, the struggle against AIDS, is also a struggle over questions of racial injustice, questions of heterosexism, questions of the way gender is constructed in the culture, questions of social justice, questions of xenophobia, questions about how the "other" is articulated in a culture. It is about how all these cultural boundaries and meanings which human beings use to define themselves, perceive each other, and, not incidentally, perpetrate injustices, enact themselves in the machinery of one little virus. And this means that solving the problems associated with that one little virus forces us to confront all these other issues.

AIDS in fact connects to almost everything. So if you want to tackle AIDS you need at least to engage, if not actually to tackle, these larger questions of social justice. That, of course, is precisely what's been going on for years now in the much-publicized struggles over HIV. Indeed, struggles over these larger issues have been one of the most striking features of "the HIV movement." The interconnections which AIDS forces into view carry us back to what I have called liberal education as education for human freedom.

My own bias in this, the lesson I've already urged upon you, is to view HIV/AIDS and even health itself as means to an end rather than as ends in themselves. Our larger goal is not to make sure that students know about HIV/AIDS, but that they leave our institutions as engaged, empowered citizens who think of themselves as having a self-conscious relationship and an obligation to a larger community—the community in which they will live their civic and social lives.

This is not just because engagement, empowerment, and community are important in and of themselves, although I certainly think they are. Closer to home for the theme of HIV/AIDS, I think that engagement, empowerment, and community are our best assurance that students will engage health care seriously both while attending college and when they're finally out in the world. Engaged, empowered, community-connected citizens are our best defense against HIV/AIDS. Without them, the struggle against HIV/AIDS is very likely to fail altogether. Without engagement, without empowerment, without a sense of obligation across the borders that set us apart from each other and that set us against each other, there is little hope that this particular disease—or equally vicious diseases yet to come—will ever be extirpated from the human community.

QUALITIES OF THE LIBERALLY EDUCATED PERSON

So let me close, having said all of this, with the core of my thoughts about what it means to be a liberally educated person. The trouble with universities is that we rarely talk about what that pious phrase "liberal education" really means. We talk instead about requirements. Usually our requirements have almost nothing to do with liberal education in the broad sense I've urged of education for human freedom.

To get at this I'll ask the question: "How would you recognize a liberally educated person if you saw one, if you bumped into one on the street?" I mean a person whose freedom and personal growth have actually been well served by education.

I offer ten qualities. Ask yourself how they relate to the struggle over HIV/AIDS because I think that every single one of them is profoundly important to any successful engagement with this complex biological and cultural phenomenon called AIDS.

So, how would you recognize liberally educated persons?

1. *They know how to listen and to hear.* This is so simple that it probably doesn't seem worth saying, but in our distracted, over-busy age I think it's worth declaring that an educated person knows how to pay attention to people and to the world around them. They work hard to hear what other people are saying. They can follow an argument, track logical reasoning, detect illogic, hear the emotions that lie behind both the logic and the illogic, and ultimately empathize with the person who is feeling those emotions. No debate, no struggle to overcome HIV/AIDS, will happen without having the ability to hear—hear the people who oppose you, hear the people who are your allies, hear the feelings, the arguments, the ideas, the interconnections.

2. *They read and they understand.* This too is simple to say but very difficult to achieve because there are so many ways of reading in the world. An educated person is literate across a wide range of genres and media. They can enjoy reading popular fiction ranging from the latest bestseller or detective novel or comic book to a work of classic literature, and they are engaged by works of non-fiction ranging from biographies to debates about current policy to the latest discoveries of science. But skilled readers know how to read far more than just words or magazines

or books. They know how to enjoy wandering through a great art museum or are moved by what they hear in a concert hall. They recognize the extraordinary human achievements that are represented by contemporary athletes working in fields as diverse as tennis or gymnastics or football. They are engaged by classic and contemporary works of theater and cinema. They are able to see in television a valuable window on the popular culture. They can wander through a prairie or a woodland and recognize the creatures they encounter there, the meaning of the rocks, the lay of the land. They can look across a farmer's field and know the crops that they see there—recognize that those crops will eventually end up in one form or another on their own dinner table. They can appreciate good food whether they encounter it in a four-star French restaurant or in a local county fair. They recognize fine craftsmanship, whether in carpentry or plumbing or auto mechanics. They can surf the World Wide Web. They can read the *Journal of the American Medical Association* and they can also watch *Angels in America*. And they can find, in radically different forms of discourse such as these, crucial and equally valuable insights into the meaning of HIV/AIDS. For an educated person, all of these are special forms of reading, profound ways in which the eyes and the ears, and the other senses become attuned to the infinite wonders and talents that make up the human and the natural world. As with the other items on this list of mine, none of us can possibly attain full competence in all of these ways of reading. But the mark of an educated person is to be competent in many of them and curious about all of them. Encountering the world as a fascinating and extraordinarily intricate set of texts waiting to be read and understood—surely this is one of the most important marks of an educated person.

3. *They can talk with anyone.* An educated person knows how to talk. They can give a speech. They can make people laugh. They can ask thoughtful questions and they can hold a conversation with anyone they meet, whether that person is a high school dropout or a Nobel Laureate, a child or a patient in a hospital, a factory worker or a farmer or a corporate CEO, a patient dying of AIDS, an FDA bureaucrat, a scientist reporting on the latest findings concerning protein sheaths. All of these are people one can talk with and understand. Moreover, educated persons participate in such conversations not because they like to talk about themselves, but because they are genuinely interested in the other person. A friend of mine says that one of the most important things his father ever told him was that in having a conversation his job was "to figure out what's so neat about what the other person does." It would be hard to imagine a more succinct description of this key quality of an educated person.

4. *They can write clearly and persuasively and movingly.* What goes for talking goes for writing as well. An educated person knows the fine craft of putting words on paper. I'm not talking about the ability to parse a sentence or compose a paragraph or write an essay. I mean the ability to express what is in your mind and in your heart so as to get these things across to the person who reads your words so as to teach, persuade, and move that person. I'm talking about writing as a form of touching—akin to the touching that happens in a wonderfully exhilarating conversation.

5. *They can solve a wide variety of puzzles and problems.* This ability to solve puzzles and problems bespeaks many other skills. These include basic numeracy, an ability to handle numbers and see that many problems which appear to turn on questions of quality can in fact often be reinterpreted as questions of quantity. These days a comparable skill involves the ability to run a computer, whether for word processing, or doing taxes, or playing games. I could go on but the broader and more practical skills I'm describing here are those of the analyst, the manager, the engineer, the critic: the ability to look at a complicated reality, break it into pieces, figure out how it works, with the end result of being able to do practical things in the real world. Part of that challenge, of course, is the ability to put reality back together again after you've broken it down into pieces. This is just as important as the act of breaking the world into pieces, even though we often forget the need to put it back together again. For only by putting the world back together again can we accomplish our practical goals without violating the integrity of the world we're trying to change. In the world of HIV/AIDS, this means remembering that the patient, the medical problem in the bed in front of you, is also a person, a person with a whole life, in which the status of being defined as "patient" is only one tiny subset of the whole.

6. *Educated people respect rigor, not so much for its own sake, but as a way of seeking truth.* This is to say, truly educated people love learning, but they love wisdom more. They can appreciate a closely reasoned argument without being unduly impressed by mere logic. They understand that knowledge always serves values and they strive to put these two, knowledge and values, into constant dialogue with each other. The ability to recognize true rigor is one of the most important achievements in any education, but it is worthless, even dangerous, if it is not placed also in the service of some larger vision that renders it also humane. Medicine without a vision of health, and knowledge of disease without attention to wellness, all too easily become destructive of the very ends that they seek to serve.

7. *They practice respect and humility, tolerance, and self-criticism.* This is another way of saying that they can feel and understand the power of other people's dreams and nightmares as well as their own. They have the intellectual range and the emotional generosity to step outside their own experiences and prejudices to recognize the parochialism of their own viewpoints, thereby opening themselves to perspectives very different from their own. This quality of intellectual openness and tolerance is among the most important values we associate with liberal education. It is impossible to imagine the struggle against HIV/AIDS without that commitment to tolerance. It's hard to imagine a more important core value that needs reinforcing if the struggle is to succeed. From this commitment to tolerance, flow all those aspects of liberal learning that celebrate the value of learning foreign languages, exposing oneself to cultures far distant from one's own, learning the history of long-ago times, and encountering the many ways in which men and women have known the sacred and given names to their gods. From a deep encounter with history and geography and culture comes a rich sense of how very different people are from each other and how much they also share in common.

8. *They understand how to get things done in the world.* In describing the goals of his Rhodes scholarship, Cecil Rhodes spoke of trying to identify young people who would spend their lives engaged in what he called "the world's fight," by which he meant the struggle to leave the world a better place than one finds it. Learning how to get things done in the world in an effort to leave it a better place is surely one of the most practical and important lessons we can take from any education. It is fraught with peril because the power to act in the world can so easily be abused. But we fool ourselves if we think we can avoid acting, avoid exercising power, avoid joining the world's fight. Not to act is to abandon to others our own responsibility to try to make the world a better place even in the face of what we know to be injustice. And so we study power and ask ourselves what it means to act rightly and wrongly in our use of power. We struggle to try to know how we can do good and avoid doing wrong. We deploy our power to defeat a virus and defeat too the ways our own culture adds to the burdens of those who carry it.

9. *They nurture and empower the people around them.* One of the most important things that tempers the exercise of power and shapes right action is surely the recognition that no one ever acts alone. A liberally educated person understands that they belong to a community whose prosperity and well-being are crucial to their own and they help that community flourish by giving of themselves to make the success of others possible. If we speak of education for freedom, then one of

the crucial insights of a liberal education must be that the freedom of the individual is only possible in a free community, and vice versa. It is the community that empowers the free individual just as it is free individuals who lead and empower the community. Individuals have made great contributions to the fight against HIV/AIDS, but any progress they have made has inevitably taken place in the context of a much larger culture and community that empowered the work they did. The fulfillment of high talent, the just exercise of power, the celebration of human diversity: Nothing so redeems these things as the recognition that what seem like personal triumphs are in fact the achievements of our common humanity.

10. *They follow E.M. Forster's injunction in the novel* Howard's End*: "Only connect."* More than anything else, being an educated person means being able to see connections so as to be able to make sense of the world and act within it in creative ways. All of the other qualities that I've just described—listening, reading, writing, talking, puzzle-solving, seeing the world through others' eyes, empowering others, leading—every last one of these things is finally about connecting. A liberal education is about gaining the power and the insight and the generosity and finally the freedom and the wisdom to connect. If one could pick just one phrase that would answer the question of what it means to be a liberally educated person surely this would be it: Only connect. And I would also argue I can imagine no better way of fighting HIV/AIDS than the same phrase: Only connect. It's the core project. Without it, all else fails.

Education for human freedom also means education for human community. The two cannot exist without each other. Every one of the ten qualities I have just described is a craft or skill or way of being in the world that frees us to act with greater knowledge, greater power. But each of these ten qualities also makes us ever more aware of the connections we have with other people and with the rest of the planet. So they remind us of the obligations we have to use our knowledge and our power responsibly, generously, caringly.

If I'm right that all of these qualities are finally about connecting, then we need to confront one last paradox about liberal education. In the act of making us free, it also binds us to the communities that gave us our freedom in the first place. It makes us responsible to those communities in a way that limits our freedom. In the end, it turns out that liberty is not about thinking or saying or doing whatever we want. It is about exercising our freedom in such a way as to make the world a better place, not just for ourselves, but for everyone and everything around us.

So we remember those two words of E.M. Forster's, "Only connect." I've said that they are as good an answer as any I know to what it means to be a liberally educated person. But they are also as good a description as any I know for the most powerful and generous form of human connection that we call love. The love I mean here is not romantic or passionate love, but the love that lies at the heart of all the great human religious traditions. Liberal education nurtures human freedom in the service of human community, which is to say that, in the end, it nurtures and celebrates love. Whether we speak of our schools or our universities or ourselves, whether we speak of education or the fight against HIV/AIDS, I hope we will hold fast to this as our constant practice in the full depth of its richness and many meanings. I hope we will nurture and celebrate love. I hope we will "only connect."

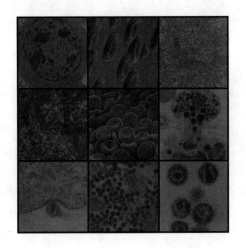

FOUR

HIV/AIDS IN THE ACADEMY:

ENGAGEMENT AND LEARNING IN A CONTEXT OF CHANGE

Richard P. Keeling, M.D.
UNIVERSITY OF WISCONSIN

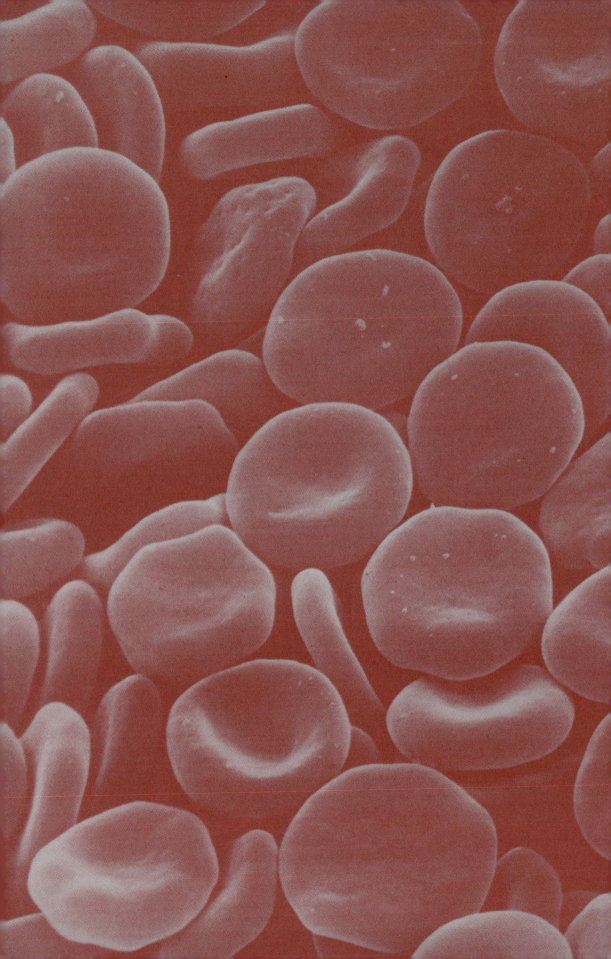

Four important ideas define the framework of this discussion:

- Attention to complex, challenging health issues, and HIV/AIDS in particular, strengthens the relationship of colleges and universities to their students in regard to health, learning, and citizenship, and it can improve outcomes in each area.

- Fruitful discussion of HIV/AIDS and other pressing public health concerns requires engagement across academic disciplines and integration among the traditionally separate structures of academic and student affairs.

- Better HIV/AIDS prevention requires a focus not only on scientific facts and epidemiologic data, but also on essential, deeper human questions about the self, relationships, community, culture, and the obligations and responsibilities of individuals and societies; the scholarly, intellectual resources of higher education are vital to exploring those questions.

- Improving health (in any community, including college campuses, and for all individuals, including college students) demands thinking of health in collective terms, as community property; understanding the social and cultural contexts of health and health decisions; and allocating resources toward community-based, rather than purely individual, interventions.

COLLEGES AND UNIVERSITIES RESPOND TO HIV/AIDS

The epidemic of HIV/AIDS has never been entirely—or even primarily—experienced anywhere as an episode in the biological relationship between microorganisms and human beings. It has been, instead, a series of events that have, taken together, illuminated the nature and character of relationships among people, from the small scale of human bonds and intimacies to the framing of diplomatic and economic balances between nations. HIV produces, of course, an infectious disease; its encounter with human immune systems is classically unforgiving, and its legacy of disability, death, and loss is unforgettable. But to understand HIV/AIDS in clinical, virological, or statistical terms alone is to miss its fundamental meanings, and to overlook its broad significance as a problem in our common health, our sense of community, and our politics. This is not to say that the concrete, ground-level realities of HIV/AIDS (sickness and death) are unimportant by themselves; rather, the place of HIV/AIDS in culture, history, and modem society adds symbols and meaning to the experience of each person, family, or community coping with its presence. Those layers of meaning deeply affect how a person living with HIV interprets, knows, and describes the experience, and they influence how that person is seen, cared for, and served.

The fact that HIV is transmitted by blood and certain body fluids, and especially its position as a sexually transmitted disease, make its biology a social, and even political, concern. Its known or perceived associations with injected illegal drugs, shared needles, gay and bisexual men, cities, and relationships not usually covered under the umbrella of "traditional family values" have made HIV/AIDS, and the people affected, seem not just different but alien, dark, sinister, and frightening. As the epidemic evolves, it centers ever more clearly on people at the margins of society; the guiding currents of its course are inequities of socioeconomic status, class, race, and gender. Dealing with HIV/AIDS as a critical problem in personal and public health requires attention to all of the complex, interrelated social, cultural, and political issues that those inequities define—and to the murky uncertainties of attitudes, beliefs, and behaviors that cloud our understanding of sexuality.

Our adjustments to and management of the problems caused by HIV/AIDS have revealed hard facts about difference, prejudice, and suffering. Understanding the impact of this epidemic requires thinking seriously about the distribution of wealth, inequities in access to health care, the deterioration of inner cities, the unsolved problems of race, and the availability of treatment on demand for people who use intravenous drugs. It is impossible to trace the path of HIV/AIDS through the American mind, heart, and spirit without examining its connections to sex, gender, sexual orientation, love, passion, illness, and death. A person who says "I have AIDS" makes multiple disclosures and runs multiple risks. "I have AIDS" means a great deal more than "I have an acquired immune deficiency disorder, caused by a virus." It is still true that a diagnosis of HIV/AIDS "says" more about who you are—and what you do, or did—than what you have.

As is the case in society more generally, the history of higher education's attempts to comprehend and respond to HIV/AIDS is a complex record of desperate fear, great courage, terrible confusion, and real clarity. Initially, informal networks of concerned students, faculty, and staff arose in response to the concrete realities of need and fear: someone was infected, or sick, and something must be done to help and protect. In parallel (but usually not in relation), institutions established formal structures (task forces, committees, strategic plans, policies) to manage risks, satisfy constituents, and define courses of action. The informal groups worked hard on individual problems and sought to insert gentleness in the policies and programs that task forces developed.

Over time, the protections devised by formal committees began to seem unnecessary, and the detailed, algorithmic policies were seldom used. Most of the predicted crises in classrooms, residence halls, and recreational facilities did not materialize, nor did the anticipated expansion of the epidemic among privileged, white, heterosexual students. HIV/AIDS began to seem ordinary. Many of the people who came together to serve friends "burned out," moved on to work elsewhere, or, sick themselves, died. On most campuses, dedicated HIV/AIDS peer education programs faded away as the epidemic left the front page and turned up mostly among the urban poor, people of color, and certain groups of gay and bisexual men. No significant presence of students with HIV emerged on most campuses. The once diverting, entertaining "safer sex" and condom distribution programs got old and predictable. Students began to seem merely bored by "AIDS talks," and HIV/AIDS drifted to their proverbial back burner. Most students now feel that HIV/AIDS is clearly not a personal threat to them.

Graduates, however, must cope with a world that has suffered much, and will suffer far more, from HIV/AIDS. They will interact with people who have HIV/AIDS as citizens, employers, co-workers, relatives, partners in sexual relationships, managers, neighbors, and leaders. They will encounter repeatedly the key issues that the epidemic highlights: inequity, race, class, poverty, access, participation, sexuality. They will bear responsibility for better prevention programs for the generations that follow them and for providing humane services to persons (and their families, of all kinds) living with HIV/AIDS. Some of those graduates will work in the global marketplace, trade in multiple languages, or influence the politics of international relations. HIV/AIDS will be a terrible factor in the world's business, wars, and relief efforts. All of our graduates must be prepared to make ethical decisions, establish relationships, and develop community as participating citizens. Regardless of the presence or absence of any specific intrusion of HIV/AIDS into their personal or family lives, this epidemic will be, in fact, a critical issue in the world they inherit and, therefore, a problem for all of them.

EPIDEMIOLOGY AND CULTURAL ECOLOGY OF HIV/AIDS ON CAMPUS

Studies of the patterns of infection with HIV among college and university students confirm, more or less, students' perceptions about the epidemic's biological relationship to them. Most students would probably say that (1) HIV/AIDS is an important public health issue but not a significant or frequent problem on campus and not a risk for them personally; (2) most people they know of who have HIV/AIDS are not students, and they can't think of any students they know who have HIV; and (3) if they do know any students who have HIV/AIDS, those affected students are gay or bisexual men.

Two nationwide research projects conducted between 1988 and 1992 found that approximately 0.2 percent of students (about 1 in 500) have HIV as determined by positive antibody tests. There has been no national study of the prevalence of HIV among college and university students since then, but other indicators do not suggest that there is any convincing reason to think this number has increased significantly. Rates of diagnosis of other sexually transmitted diseases or unwanted pregnancies among students have not increased since 1992 (and, in fact, some such measures show a decrease). Tests of the frequency of HIV infection among new recruits for military service have showed stable or declining rates. The experience of campus health centers does not suggest either (1) an increasing number of positive antibody tests among students, or (2) a greater frequency of clinical or counseling services provided to students with HIV/AIDS. HIV antibody counseling and testing services in college settings mostly test a very low-risk population of the unnecessarily "worried well." At the same time, of course, other seroepidemiologic surveys and health department reports demonstrate a progressively greater presence of HIV among people of color, and especially women (and most especially, women and children in poverty). The pattern of HIV/AIDS among college students is very different.

Taken together, the two reliable studies of the prevalence of HIV among college students showed that students were far more likely to be infected with HIV if they were male, older than 25, and enrolled in a large institution with more than 25,000 students. While both studies identified women with HIV, there were few, and the prevalence of HIV among college women was tiny as compared to the prevalence among men. We know from other investigations that very few college students, male or female, are injecting drug users; given that, the fact that the great majority of infected students are male (and the reality that, in heterosexual relationships, women are at greater risk for infection than men) strongly suggests that most students with HIV were infected by sexual contact with other men. Neither of the national research studies specifically asked students to disclose their sexual orientation, so this conclusion cannot be definitively proven by the existing data. However, it is certainly consistent with the data and with the experience of college and university health services over the past decade. The great majority of students with HIV/AIDS are, and have been, gay and bisexual men.

The paradigm of universal risk ("anyone can be infected"; "it's not who you are, it's what you do"; "AIDS is not a gay disease") swept campuses in the late 1980's. Legitimate uncertainty about the future course of the epidemic permitted HIV/AIDS to be wrapped into campus-wide health education programs with the intent of reaching—and changing the behavior of—every student. Since every student was theoretically at risk, colleges and universities could remove most of the emphasis on gay concerns, and, in the process, subtract exactly the elements of HIV/AIDS prevention that made it most controversial. As was true everywhere else, it was the connections, associations, and perceptions associated with HIV/AIDS—not its microbiology—that created discomfort. By disconnecting the epidemic from homosexuality (usually done unintentionally or, if not, at least with good motives) colleges could sustain health promotion programs, recruit and retain peer educators, and conduct campus-wide "safer sex" programs—none of which would have been acceptable on most campuses if their focus had been risk reduction for gay and bisexual men. By the middle of the 1990's, though, the idea of universal risk had lost power and credibility, and students' (correct) perceptions about the real campus epidemiology of HIV began to reinforce their loss of personal interest in the epidemic. Culture moves on; more than ten years after HIV/AIDS became a campus issue, some institutions began to be able to do what they could not do earlier and developed specific HIV/AIDS prevention programs for gay and bisexual male students, just as efforts based on universal risk were fading.

Just as HIV/AIDS seems a problem of "the other" in our culture, then, it increasingly seems so on campus. HIV/AIDS seems marginal; it "lives" off campus, mostly, and it affects people whose lives are mysterious to most students. Most students, faculty, and staff who have, or have died from, HIV/AIDS are different, too, because of their sexual orientation. And, actually, people in the college community who have HIV/AIDS are more likely by far to be faculty or staff than students—an observation that further distances most students from the epidemic, even when it does appear close to their own lives. In many ways, then, students' common observations about the impact of the epidemic on campus are right.

Though this analysis itself will frighten or frustrate some dedicated students, faculty, and staff who have fought hard to keep HIV/AIDS alive as a campus issue, it is not the analysis itself that should cause alarm. Rather, we must all attend to the meaning we choose to place on the facts. The danger lies in deciding that HIV/AIDS is not a problem for students, or not a problem for colleges and universities—in taking reassurance from the facts, rather than concern; in looking narrowly at the here-and-now for students and institutions. The questions are these: if AIDS does not pose an immediate threat of disease to most students, does that mean it is not important for colleges and universities to address it? And if HIV/AIDS primarily endangers certain "others," does that mean it is not important for all of us to attend to it? Does the fact that HIV/AIDS primarily affects students who are men who have sex with men alter the way a college should respond?

There are fundamental, critical reasons for colleges, universities, and communities to work very hard in responding to the issues, concerns, and needs created by HIV/AIDS, no matter what the specifics of its epidemiology are at any particular time.

- Regardless of the question of personal risk, HIV/AIDS is an important social, cultural, and global problem that demands the attention of every student, school, community, and society. Responding to problems that primarily affect other people is basic to citizenship and community.

- Education about HIV/AIDS is education for life. Our graduates will work, manage, and lead in a complex society; they will have to handle concerns about HIV/AIDS in a variety of settings and roles, and they should be prepared to think and decide carefully. Learning about HIV/AIDS will prepare them to deal with a great many other complex human issues.

- HIV/AIDS forces us to confront very difficult questions of difference, diversity, prejudice, and inequity—not only within American society, but across nations. These are issues that must be faced in an increasingly diverse society and an increasingly integrated, multinational culture.

- HIV/AIDS demands a clear focus on issues of inclusion that bear not only on social and health problems but also on critical thinking. Post-modem epistemology, feminist thought, and challenges to the "western canon" are not just academic issues; they will be infused in the way graduates work, think, and learn in the future.

- Our students will graduate into a shrinking world with permeable international boundaries, global markets, and shared health problems.

- HIV/AIDS is emblematic of the problem of new emerging global infectious diseases, most of them viral (e.g., Ebola virus, Hantavirus); understanding their patterns and coping with their impact will be essential for 21st century citizens.

- The patterns of HIV/AIDS among most students are not illustrative of the whole epidemic. There are multiple "subepidemics" within the larger one, and, in some populations and communities, HIV continues to be devastating. Some students, particularly if they are non-traditional, urban, returning adults, live and work in those deeply affected communities. To ignore HIV/AIDS is to neglect critical realities of those students' lives.

- The pattern documented in the two national studies, and supported by subsequent indirect observations and campus experience, is only a "snapshot" of one small element of the epidemic of HIV/AIDS, taken at one point in time. Though current indicators do not suggest that the pattern is changing substantially, alterations in relationships and student demographics may produce a very different picture in the future.

- Finally, gay and bisexual male students matter, too. Despite much social progress, it is still necessary to state the obvious: noticing that HIV/AIDS primarily affects gay and bisexual men on campus does not reduce its importance to colleges and universities. Writing HIV/AIDS off as "just a gay problem" is an inhumane, wrong-headed response. Institutions of higher education should be concerned not only about the needs of gay and bisexual men, and not only about the broader needs of gay, lesbian, bisexual, and transgender students, but also about the specific relationship of gay and bisexual men to HIV. That is, schools should be interested in what it means that most students (and faculty and staff) with HIV/AIDS are gay and bisexual men. What does that say about homophobia, and support for same-sex relationships, and the safety of "coming out" on campus, or in society? What does it teach about the intersecting questions of gender, sexuality, biology, and culture in determining behavior?

Responding to the problems of HIV/AIDS, then, demands leadership and perspective —a vision beyond the immediate presence and visibility of the epidemic on campuses at any moment.

PREVENTION, PUBLIC HEALTH, AND THE UNDERSTANDING OF HIV/AIDS

Students, becoming citizens, are all going to have to deal with HIV/AIDS; in doing so, they will have to manage very complex issues in both personal and "public" domains. This same attention to complicated issues defines the return of "public health" and "prevention" to their most noble and important roots in assessing and solving important social problems.

The great challenge to support for public health programs is that when they work, nothing happens, or, at least, nothing bad happens. Historically, public health arose in response to certain disasters and was then held accountable for the occurrence of other ones. Long before there were sophisticated scientific or epidemiologic tools, public health looked into the roots of human tragedies—sickness and death—with a careful, holistic social analysis. More than a century ago, public health practitioners (many of whom were nurses) knew nothing about what had not been discovered—say, cryptosporidium—but they knew a great deal about the effects of drinking contaminated water. They had no devices with which to define the safe level of bacteria in streams, but they knew that clean water was a public health priority. In trying to improve health, they worked to make clean water, sanitary housing, and decent food and shelter available; they centered their efforts among the poor and marginalized citizens in evolving urban communities. They did not differentiate pressing health concerns from social issues; poverty was both a social problem and a health concern, because of its many consequences in the quality of life.

It is also important that, at its roots, public health was not concerned with "personal wellness"; the Hull House in Chicago preceded the Battle Creek Sanitarium both in concept and in fact. The Hull House Settlement confronted disease and death among the urban poor by providing safe shelter, clean water, and food; the Battle Creek "San" housed Dr. Charles H. Kellogg's attempt to achieve immortality for himself and his patients by vegetarian diets, exercise, and a panoply of bowel regimens. Public health went where people lived to do its work; Kellogg and a host of successors have taken them out of their usual environments to be "well." Personal wellness was both a literal and a philosophical abstraction.

Public health strategies have seldom intersected with the lives of the privileged. The residents of Hull House had no hope of going to Battle Creek for wellness, and the wealthy (but, sadly, not immortal) clients of the "San" would never have thought of poverty as a health issue. Bad water and unsanitary living conditions were, and seemed, very distant from their lives—and so did public health. In modem society, a kind of dichotomy arose between poverty/public health and privilege/wellness; wellness programs and ideas (fitness, personal trainers, coronary risk reduction, etc.) were the options (and, in some groups, the perceived obligations) of individuals, and they paid very little attention to contexts, social problems, and culture. The public health department took care of the social and venereal diseases of the poor; people who could afford private medical care did not go there.

Meanwhile, public health programs, with more elegant tools and quantitative capacities, focused increasingly on counting, tracking, and data collection. What was wrong with contaminated water or bad air could now be specified with impressive precision. The path of a contagious disease through a community could be portrayed— and, eventually, predicted—with accuracy. Who smoked cigarettes, and when they started, and what happened to them when they did, or who had which sexually transmitted diseases, or how many adolescent women had unwanted pregnancies—all could be answered. The concepts of "risk factors" and "risk behaviors" were well in place by the time HIV/AIDS arrived, so the epidemic could be measured, graphed, and explained—to a point. That point is defined by asking not just what, or how many, but why.

Why was HIV/AIDS happening? Unfortunately, of course, counting the cases did not explain what was really going on, and public health was initially "out of practice" in asking fundamental human questions. Whether sexually transmitted or passed through shared needles, the spread of HIV has a relational character; it occurs in the complex lives of humans as unpredictable social animals surrounded by societies and cultures with traditions and customs. But the first decade of responses was dominated by uncomplicated, individually focused, wellness-type messages like "just say no" and "always use a condom." And now public health and prevention must confront an epidemic that continues despite the presence of high levels of basic protective knowledge and the easy availability of prevention resources, like condoms. Knowing how many new HIV infections there are among, say, young gay men does not help much, except for knowing where to aim with some better prevention message; we must know why.

Asking why behavior does not change, or why certain patterns of disease happen as they do among certain populations, returns public health to its roots. Asking why demands attention to the contexts of behavior, the social conditions underlying disease, and the cultural context itself. Asking why extends the traditional triad of prevention (primary, secondary, and tertiary) by adding another dimension.

- Tertiary prevention attempts to prevent the complications (such as death) of an established disease. In AIDS, tertiary prevention focuses on treating the opportunistic infections or cancers that develop in people with severe immunodeficiency.

- Secondary prevention tries to prevent the development of disease among people who already have the risk factors for that disease. In the case of HIV/AIDS, this means treating people who have HIV with medications to try to prevent them from developing AIDS itself.

- Primary prevention means keeping people from acquiring the risk factors for the disease in the first place; regarding HIV/AIDS, this means preventing new HIV infections (sexual abstinence, safer sex, condoms, clean needles, etc.).

- Community-based prevention—the new element—looks beyond primary prevention to identify the social and cultural forces that expose people to risk factors, and then attempts to prevent those exposures.

Community based, or "contextual," prevention, has an environmental focus; it asks why risk factors are present. Primary prevention stops, in the case of tobacco abuse, at encouraging teenagers not to start smoking; it provides a series of self-defense strategies, limits sales of the product, and educates children about the health consequences of smoking. Community based prevention, on the other hand, goes farther: it asks why teenagers start smoking in the first place, and that question leads to explorations of tobacco advertising, cigarette promotions at major events, and the psychology of adolescence. Community based prevention forces a political analysis and it uses political tools—regulation, legal challenges, media attention.

Community based prevention also asks difficult questions and suggests challenging solutions when we apply it to HIV/AIDS:

- *Why* young people take risks in sexual relationships leads to a complex social analysis of advertising messages, role models, the establishment of "adolescence" as a developmental phase, the declining influence of traditional religions, changes in family structures, and the "get it now" assumptions of consumer culture. Turning children and adolescents into consumers is directly related to the spread of HIV.

- *Why* people who have more than adequate information about HIV and know how to protect themselves still get infected opens up a wide array of further questions about the translation of knowledge into behavior, all of them filtered through culture and context. These questions are pertinent, for example, to young gay and bisexual men (including those in college), and the answers, if pursued diligently, will open further inquiries into the effects of homophobia on the development of committed relationships among men who have sex with men, the influence of genetic or biological "imperatives" in male sexual behavior, and the absence of attractive, realistic role models.

- *Why* women of color in poverty have increasing rates of HIV infection leads rapidly to an analysis of gender, power in relationships, the impact of poverty on sexual behavior, the reasons for persistent poverty, and the different accountabilities of individual, partners, community, and the public for behavior and its outcomes.

To understand the epidemic of HIV/AIDS without asking questions like those is to miss the point entirely. HIV/AIDS is no more just a sexually transmitted disease to be counted and tracked than murder is just a problem in ballistics. Yes, the bullet caused the death—but preventing murder demands an understanding of why the gun was fired. Answering all the questions that HIV/AIDS asks will require genuinely complex thinking; it will demand the resources not just of virologists, immunologists, epidemiologists, and clinicians, but also the ideas of anthropologists, sociologists, psychologists, economists, and historians. Dealing effectively with HIV/AIDS will require bringing into the discussion writers, poets, and artists who can understand, explain, and express in new ways the most deeply human questions and issues that sexuality, sickness, alienation, and death stimulate.

Better HIV/AIDS prevention then needs critical thinking, an interdisciplinary perspective, and careful analysis. It also requires courage and rigor; hard questions and controversial answers are inevitable. Both the questions and the answers will lead to discussion and debate about fundamental social problems. Just as HIV/AIDS then illuminates pressing social and cultural realities, preventing the further spread of the epidemic will require understanding those realities, deciphering their influence on individuals and their behavior, and attempting societal solutions. Attention to HIV/AIDS in the academy promises the opportunity to prepare students to think carefully through public issues (whether or not they are directly related to health) as they arise. And colleges and universities provide a magnificent diversity of forums (from classrooms to residence halls, newspapers, cafes, community service projects, and student organizations, to name only a few) for that preparation. The intellectual capital of institutions of higher education thus becomes a resource in service of broader, deeper views of prevention.

HEALTH AS COMMUNITY PROPERTY, THE CHALLENGE OF CITIZENSHIP

The preceding discussion properly implies an understanding of "health" that challenges both the prevailing view in our culture and the organization of health care on campuses and in our society. We think most often of health as a biomedical quality possessed by individuals and measured through the use of a variety of scientific parameters; indeed, we use modifiers to specify some other kind of health than that (e.g., public health, community health, mental health). The certification of health, in fact, is usually provided by medical professionals after they assess certain characteristics of a person as compared with norms derived from data collected from representative members of the population. Health is then measured in individual terms. Similarly, we think of health behaviors as purely individual decisions, and we try to modify them by asking individuals to make personal changes (e.g., "just say no," or "know when to say when"). This emphasis on individuals allies our view of health much more with Kellogg and the sanitarium than with public health and Hull House. It implies that health is under one's own entire control.

A deeper analysis of health behavior, though, suggests that health and health decisions always occur in context—within a social and cultural framework experienced through traditions, customs, folkways, media messages, peer group norms, and economic realities. To say that we cannot fully comprehend HIV/AIDS without studying its connections to societal issues such as race, class, and gender is to say that we cannot understand the HIV/AIDS-related behaviors of individuals without studying the social and cultural contexts of those behaviors; both statements allude to a view of health that integrates, rather than separates, the individual members of human communities. Sexual behavior has both an exuberant, colorful, provocative context in our public media, and a repressive, cold framework of societal traditions and norms. Although people of good will might argue forcefully about the values transmitted in advertising, religious doctrines, or modern American politics, at least it seems clear that all of those factors, and many others, create pressures that influence sexual decision-making (and most other health behaviors, from alcohol and other drug use to choices about nutrition and exercise). The way college and university students drink alcohol is certainly not determined just by their personal knowledge of its chemistry and physiological effects, but rather by the complex interplay of campus traditions, peer group norms, developmental stages, and student culture. How a young woman eats is affected not only by what she knows about food groups, calories, and fat grams, but also by images of women in advertising, attitudes among both men and women she knows about what makes a woman attractive, and social norms concerning pleasure and control.

For college and university students, these issues of health behavior are, without doubt, the most pressing and important health concerns. The episodic minor illnesses and injuries that cause most visits to campus health centers are far less significant (in terms of quality of life, long-term survival, and effect on academic success) than drinking, sexual behavior, violence, and problems in eating. Most of these behaviors are deeply embedded in an internal framework of psychological health, emotions, and mood states, as well. Another way to think about these points is to recognize that the most critical health problems of students are usually not medical problems. This same point is pertinent at several other stages of life, but most pressing for youth.

To suggest that many (and, among students, most) health problems are not primarily biological and that the determinants of those problems have collective roots is to redefine health in social, cultural, and community terms. Doing so does not abolish the concept of individual responsibility, nor does it relieve individuals of accountability for their choices. It does, however, change our focus. If health is a collective property, then it is also a community responsibility. If many of the factors that influence health are social and cultural, then the behavior of communities (and society more generally) is a health concern. Instead of directing all our health resources to encouraging individual behavior change (as if individuals make isolated decisions and have complete personal control), we should then allocate resources toward understanding and influencing the "behavior" of groups —communities and cultures. We begin to design systematic, rather than individual solutions; we imagine collective, rather than just personal, action.

The challenge of addressing campus health problems successfully is one of finding community-based solutions. It means shifting resources and emphasis from "medical" approaches in college health services toward prevention and community health. Rather than expecting individual students to resist all the pressures of their environment and still make "healthy decisions," we accept collective responsibility for that environment and its implications, and we assume, together, accountability for change. Collaboration replaces simple individual choices. To reduce the harm caused by the pattern of episodic binge drinking, we must alter the prevailing norms, traditions, and customs that support it. Reaching a more healthy balance in the relationship between some groups of young women and the food they eat (or refuse, or restrict, or vomit) will require far more than better nutrition education. And changing risks of acquiring sexually transmitted pathogens (like HIV, but also including many others) will mean working with the social and community factors that contribute to risk-taking sexual behavior.

Such a shift toward a collective, or community-based, view of health and health behaviors requires that we develop the capacity for careful, humane analysis. It also demands patience in accepting long-term solutions and the courage to address underlying and entrenched societal problems. Understanding health takes thought, and improving it will take human connections, conversations, and community. HIV/AIDS is a specific, critical example of such a health problem, but the skills and mental flexibility required to understand it are general abilities that will help students think through all of the other health issues that will affect their lives, families, and communities. Students who learn to approach HIV/AIDS as a complex human and social problem may be able to think of poverty, threats to the environment, violence, or controversies about land use in the same textured way. Students who learn that managing the presence and effects of HIV/AIDS in their personal, vocational, or social lives demands both humane caution and a sense of shared responsibility may be more facile with the tools of citizenship. Students whose learning about HIV/AIDS exposes them to both the successes and failures of public policy, international relations, and health systems may feel more obligation to participate in the processes of a healthy democracy.

Seeing both the causes and the solutions of health problems as centered in community, or cultural, terms returns health to the realm of public responsibility, public discussion, and public health as originally defined. Doing so centers health in civic life and encourages participatory solutions.

NEW GENERATIONS OF LEARNERS, NEW STRUCTURES TO SUPPORT LEARNING

This reframing of health makes "health" itself a kind of interdisciplinary bridge, while, at the same time, placing it in the public, civic sphere and locating it within the shaping forces of culture. Such an adjustment recognizes, too, the identities, images, and "locations" of today's college and university students as people who learn in an integrated, interdisciplinary, public way—and reinforces current changes in the programs, agencies, and divisions that serve students on campuses. In this section, we explore the congruence of those themes with trends in understanding and preventing HIV/AIDS.

Emerging generations of college students live and learn in context, just as they experience health and make health decisions contextually (in the public, civic sphere, and within the shaping forces of culture). Unlike many generations of their predecessors, they are integrated learners. Students now bring into the academic space—classrooms, laboratories, discussion sections, lecture halls, and libraries—all of their own experience (regardless of any formal definition of what was "educational") and personal history, as well as what they have learned, often informally, from—to cite only a few examples—entertainers, the mass media, popular music, and peers. The influence of modern electronic technologies, from cable television to the Internet, has been to "democratize" learning by opening channels of access to a much broader array of sources that compete for attention, credibility, and respect. The World Wide Web has become exactly that, a global support structure that permits "network" to become a verb with meanings both active and passive.

The intellectual challenge of postmodernism, with its emphasis on the relativity of truth, knowledge, and standards in the variable contexts of a diversity of cultures, settings, and timeframes, has a very concrete, grounded representation on today's campuses. No longer is the professor the only—or necessarily the most credible—source of information. And if that professor insists on abstracting knowledge from life experience—segregating students' intellects from their bodies, relationships, emotions—students will likely downplay the importance, relevance, and pertinence of what is taught. Learning in context is, then, integrative; the challenge is not getting enough material, but rather sorting the value, importance, and strength of different "inputs." This challenge to critical thinking and analysis applies equally to the content of educational material and the development of citizenship. Figuring out the relative strength of points of view, arguments, and persuasive voices matters as much in daily community interactions (politics, advertising, consumer behavior, family life) as in any academic discourse. Connecting this point to concern about HIV/AIDS is important. Graduates of our colleges will need to make personal, professional, behavioral, and social choices about HIV/AIDS in a complex context; to do so they must integrate information and perspectives from many sources, perform a critical analysis, and decide what to do, whom to support, and what resources to deploy. The questions are not so simple, but just as concrete, as whether to trust a potential sexual partner; they will determine how public funds flow to needle exchange programs, whether middle and high school teachers can talk about condoms in classes, and if gay and lesbian couples can marry. Precisely those kinds of questions can stimulate the search for a critical analysis of competing views; the skills so learned apply broadly to many other topics, issues, and debates.

Supporting better student learning in the combined interest of education and citizenship challenges the traditional forms and patterns of higher education. Fundamental shifts in the relationship between students and institutions are clear in the evolution of learning models that substitute newly defined and demonstrated learning outcomes (such as portfolios, outcome data, or community service certification) for traditional indicators of teaching (such as clock or credit hours). Responding to both the reality of integrative learning (which is not just a theory, but a call for concreteness, or groundedness in education) and threats of diminishing resources, greater accountability, and competition for the best qualified students, many colleges and universities have begun reassessing, in a strategic way, the roles of student affairs and services. Opportunities for learning multiply for integrated, contextual learners. More spaces—including residence halls, student unions/student centers, and recreational facilities—serve as "classrooms." More people qualify as "educators." More events represent "teachable moments." Learning is less likely to be individual and solitary, and more likely to be noisy—even boisterous—and collective. And just as students resist separating their minds from the whole of their experience, so they protest the typical structures that segregate activities, times of the day, buildings, and programs into "student life" areas and "academic" ones.

Connecting living and learning—bringing together student life and the life of the mind—now unites our interest in HIV/AIDS with current trends in student affairs. The two intersect around an integrated approach to preparing educated people who will also be effective, participating citizens. Seeking to direct a greater proportion of resources toward "mission central" goals—especially learning—institutions now shift the emphasis in student services from "student development" and "support services" toward improving the learning environment in ways that integrate, rather than separate, student life and its programs with the academy's educational mission. Student affairs programs, therefore, have begun to reconnect across historical divisions, building bridges of cooperation and partnership with faculty: improving students' readiness to learn, working with faculty as experts about students' lives, enhancing and extending classroom experience, and integrating students' development in community with their preparation for citizenship. Given students' current risks and possibilities in relation to the epidemiology of HIV, it is probable that citizenship and its obligations will be the role in which they will most often encounter and deal with HIV/AIDS. But just as learning no longer occurs only in the academic sphere, the development of community (and, therefore, preparation for citizenship) no longer occurs only in "student life."

Responding to their own assessment that "If we are to collaborate with others in higher education to advance student learning, we need clear and concise guidelines for how to proceed," the American College Personnel Association and the National Association of Student Personnel Administrators joined to produce, in 1997, a statement of *Principles of Good Practice for Student Affairs.* The seven principles describe the field's commitments and, by implication, support new approaches to HIV/AIDS in higher education. They assert that "good practice in student affairs":

1. Engages students in active learning.

2. Helps students develop coherent values and ethical standards.

3. Sets and communicates high expectations for learning.

4. Uses systematic inquiry to improve student and institutional performance.

5. Uses resources effectively to achieve institutional mission and goals.

6. Forges educational partnerships that advance student learning.

7. Builds supportive and inclusive communities.

Colleges and universities, at the same time, have begun to explore changes in the basic foundations of teaching and learning. What does liberal education mean in today's context? How can the academy integrate the powerful, volatile forces of a multi-channel, fast-paced electronic society; the mind- and world-opening offerings of the Internet; and the content of today's flourishing debates about culture, the value of the intellect (and of intellectuals), and the principles of scholarship and teaching with the rich heritage of liberal learning? When knowledge is both politicized and democratized—when its essence is debatable, and its hierarchies are in question—how can higher education best promote both learning and citizenship?

The Association of American Colleges and Universities (AAC&U), in the first of a series of papers on "The Academy in Transition," *Contemporary Understandings of Liberal Education* (1998), engages these questions and derives an "emerging conceptualization of liberal learning" that places contemporary trends in the context of tradition. The "learning goals" identified therein emphasize themes that resonate with the rethinking now driving change in student affairs. They suggest the need for substantial renovations in many of the assumptions recently guiding higher education: disciplinarity, sharp distinctions between general education and major concentrations, and measuring learning by credits and courses. These goals can also be read as strong arguments for locating HIV/AIDS directly in the core of an institution's scholarship and teaching, on the one hand, and at the hub of its relationship with students and their lives, on the other:

- Acquiring intellectual skills or capacities

- Understanding multiple modes of inquiry and approaches to knowledge

- Developing societal, civic, and global knowledge

- Gaining self-knowledge and grounded values

- Concentration and integration of learning

In the recommendations made in *Contemporary Understandings of Liberal Education* for strategies to achieve these learning goals can be found both a clear description of new learning styles and strong encouragement to faculties to adopt more flexible, student-centered, inclusive pedagogies. It is not surprising that the recommendations also reinforce essential elements in the revisionist view of student affairs (active learning, systematic inquiry, educational partnerships, building supportive and inclusive communities):

- Collaborative inquiry
- Experiential learning
- Service learning
- Research or inquiry-based learning
- Integrative learning

Taken together, these goals and strategies for an emerging conceptualization of liberal learning respond, as do the *Principles of Good Practice for Student Affairs*, to students' needs as integrated learners, to current and future requirements for campus and community citizenship, to the refocusing of institutional missions, and to demands for evaluation, improvement, and accountability. The same goals and principles apply to the integration of health, learning, citizenship, and community that HIV/AIDS demands, and define a new, more central position for complex, unsolved health issues in the thinking, life, and mission of institutions of higher education.

FROM MARGIN TO MISSION: HIV/AIDS IN THE NEW ACADEMY

Current principles and trends in student affairs recast student affairs professionals as "student affairs educators" and center the field and its services in the mission of higher education. Likewise, the most pressing campus health concerns—alcohol, sexual relationships, stress, depression, and violence—acquire a new position of greater attention when understood as collective or community issues that demand thoughtful analysis and mutual action. Health requires prevention, which requires learning and thinking; reciprocally, learning and thinking require health, health requires community, and community requires citizenship. Preventing HIV/AIDS, not so inelegant and mechanical a matter as simplistic behavioral encouragements or condom distribution, becomes a shared enterprise of inquiry, debate, consensus, and community development. For today's generations of integrated, contextual learners, the infusion of HIV/AIDS as content (or its presence as a series of unresolved questions in courses, programs, and discussions) permits education about the virus, the epidemic, preventing transmission, and the social issues that it raises to emerge, often folded together with ideas, history, and politics. This is not to say that HIV/AIDS prevention becomes less deliberate; it simply becomes less abstracted, or segregated. And it is not to say that dedicated HIV/AIDS prevention efforts (from brochures to Web sites) have no further place—just that we should no longer focus on HIV/AIDS in isolation from everything else that is happening in students' intellectual, academic, and personal lives. HIV/AIDS moves, then, from margin to mission, from an occasional diversion in the paracurriculum to a fundamental place in the midst of the institution's thought and action. There, it serves to advance the academy's agendas, support a college's commitments to the public, and address the needs of new generations of learners.

The key to transformative education is engagement—with ideas, the intense material of a discipline, inspired creativity, art, beauty—as mediated, usually, through significant relationships. At the core of students' experience in college have always been their relationships with faculty. It is their teachers whom students traditionally most clearly remember as agents when higher education works—when it is truly transformative. Although several decades of student development literature could be read as suggesting otherwise, it is not primarily in para- or extracurricular activities that real development—transformation—most often occurs, but rather in the deep encounter of students with new ideas, possibilities, and imagination.

On the other hand, today's students no longer specify that such encounters must happen in traditional classrooms, or under the influence of a professor alone; as integrated, contextual learners, they are open to a wider spectrum of possible mentors and settings. Transformative education, however, remains as mysterious and unpredictable as ever; it is difficult, if not impossible, to anticipate what specific actions, readings, classes, events, conversations, or relationships will stimulate any individual student's evolution. Colleges and universities, then, might reasonably bring to bear all of their resources—faculty, staff, classes, buildings, architecture, grounds, events, gatherings, meeting places—in developing a web, or network, that offers to students the possibility of engagement, and, therefore, of transformation. As student affairs programs redefine themselves to support learning as a comprehensive institutional commitment, their staff and services become more accessible components of that very flexible network.

Pressing health concerns such as HIV/AIDS, fitted into various elements of such a network, serve an institution's purposes well. Attention to HIV/AIDS in different places, at different times, using any of a college's formats and structures, enables that institution to invest in its relationship with students—and not just with their minds. Students are embodiments, certainly, of ideas, the obligations of genetics, and the prescriptions of culture—but they also embody, in a more literal way, health, relationships, caring or negligence, and community. And they are, in ways that recognize the present and anticipate the future, embodiments also of the communities that sustain colleges and universities. Focusing on HIV/AIDS allows institutions of higher education to acknowledge those incarnations and to effect change in them. As a very grounded example of stresses in popular culture, citizenship, and interpersonal and international ethics, HIV/AIDS helps colleges make "building community" a matter of thought and action, as well as feelings. As the asker of fundamental human questions, HIV/AIDS also brings feelings into learning. And as an exemplar of the travails and battles around difference, HIV/AIDS involutes the reflexive concept of "political correctness," birthing instead, perhaps, genuine conversations about hard issues.

Attention to HIV/AIDS also provides a vehicle that grants some of an institution's wishes for interdisciplinarity and integration. The idea of interdisciplinary, or multidisciplinary, inquiry and endeavor seldom finds its own embodiment, especially on large campuses. But HIV/AIDS simply cannot be understood or explained except in the multiple languages of several fields, and its presence as both carnal consequence and intellectual puzzle means that only life and learning together—student affairs and academic disciplines—can deliver it whole to students, or, for that matter, to the community. As abstract as theories of health education can be, HIV prevention is never really anything but real, messy, and tangled. But as physical as HIV prevention always is, it never happens out of context.

Finally, HIV/AIDS stands, among the complex social problems facing colleges and universities, in a position of particular import. There are many other health concerns (especially when "health" is defined very broadly) that could, and probably should, deserve time in the curriculum, a place at the table the institution shares with the community, and a role in that institution's research and service. Poverty, land use, environmental hazards, socioeconomic inequality, illiteracy—on and on, are all unsolved problems that need higher education's attention. But in HIV/AIDS colleges and universities encounter at once the intricate idiosyncrasies and unfinished realities of students' lives, and the complex relationships that connect them to each other, and to culture. It is there that HIV/AIDS has a special place in higher education's priorities, at the level that connects ideas, courses, and degrees to students as whole people.

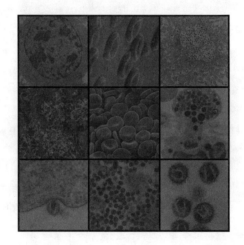

FIVE

Service Learning and HIV/AIDS Prevention:

Prospects for an Integrated Strategy

Ira Harkavy and Daniel Romer

University of Pennsylvania

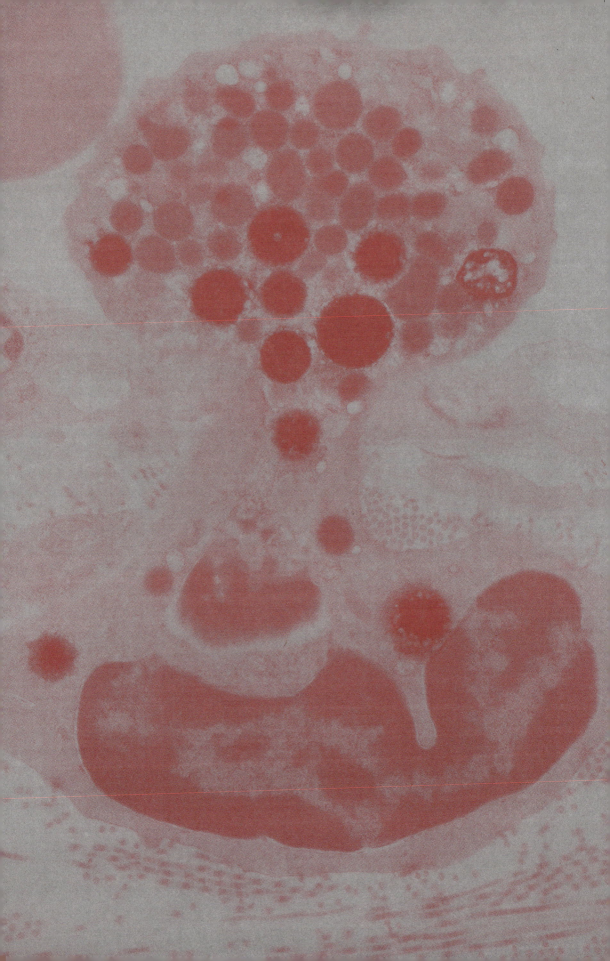

The Association of American Colleges and Universities has recommended programs to integrate HIV/AIDS prevention activities into the undergraduate curriculum. One way to do this is to incorporate service learning as both a pedagogical and action program for marshalling campus resources toward this effort. This essay provides an overview of the prospects for using service learning as an educational approach to this health problem. It argues that service learning is an appropriate vehicle for integrating pedagogy with service-oriented health promotion. However, to be effective not only in serving the needs of undergraduates and faculty but also the local community, we argue for the adoption of service learning programs that are both strategic (designed to have a measurable effect in the community) and academically based (using the best available methods of problem solving). We conclude with examples of service learning programs that illustrate the approach we advocate and provide suggestions based on this experience for others wishing to develop similar programs.

WHY THE ATTENTION TO SERVICE LEARNING?

Service learning is not a particularly new approach in higher education (Liu 1996), but it has experienced renewed attention as a possible solution to the need for greater "citizenship education" in college curricula. Along with this call is the recognition that the problems of our communities are also the problems of our campuses. There is no escaping the poverty, crime, and physical deterioration that surround many higher educational institutions. There is always the temptation to return to the mythic image of the "college on the hill" (and to suffer the consequences). But there is an increasing realization that, by becoming engaged in an effective and proactive fashion, we can contribute to the solution of these problems while also promoting the educational development of our students and faculty. Nevertheless, the reality is that no campus has developed the model for working effectively with its environment. A number of excellent experiments are underway, but they all represent partial attempts that do not mobilize the broad range of university and college resources and expertise.

In one sense, there has always been an intersection between the campus and the community, particularly as it relates to career objectives and the world of work. In that sense, service learning has evolved as a subset of the broader class of pedagogy encompassed by experiential education (Furco 1996). Included in this class are related experiences such as internships and co-operative learning. Although similar, the goals of these activities can be distinguished from service learning (Price and Martello 1996).

Internships have developed as opportunities to apply one's discipline in a career setting so that experience can be gained for future employment. Examples include placing education students in classrooms and medical students in clinics. Cooperative education can also entail placing students in the community, but, again, the emphasis lies on immediate career goals. Examples include law students taking summer positions in law firms and architecture students working part-time in architecture firms. From the perspective of the host organization, the co-op experience is an opportunity to identify new employees, while the internship experience is an opportunity to support training and, ultimately, the discipline.

Service learning, as the concept has evolved, has quite different goals. It seeks to provide experiences that lead to better citizenship, greater understanding of community needs, and help in solving social problems. Examples include undergraduate placements in local schools to develop special curricula that their faculties cannot cover (e.g., science mini-courses) or placements in community centers to assist poor families in finding work. The host organizations in these placements not only benefit from the assistance that students bring but may also gain from the insights and solutions that students contribute. The goal is not to identify new employees or to provide training for a discipline but, rather, to expose students to the problems of their communities and to encourage their involvement in finding solutions. To the degree these insights are also integrated in classroom activities and discussion, the goals of service learning are furthered even more.

Despite the good intentions associated with the goals of service learning, we remain skeptical that the activities typically involved in such approaches are sufficient for the tasks we face. For us, service learning courses, which a *NY Times* article defined as placing students "in environments in which their experiences are likely to augment their classroom work, and where they can actually do *some* good for others" [emphasis added], will not be sufficient to produce the intellectual and citizenship development needed to improve our communities and society. A much more robust approach, in which students do more than "some" good, but actually contribute to solving community problems, is required.

Partial attempts simply will not do for either higher education or society. A full-hearted and full-minded effort is needed—one that defines the problems of the community as the strategic problem for American higher education. Ernest Boyer's extraordinarily influential call for creating the "New American College" has relevance here. Deploring the "crisis in our public schools" and desperate condition of "our cities," Boyer challenged American higher educators to change radically their priorities and act effectively to meet their civic and societal responsibilities: "Do colleges really believe they can ignore social pathologies that surround schools and erode the educational foundations of our nation?" Specifically, Boyer (1994) called for creating a

> New American College.... [which takes] special pride in its capacity to connect thought to action, theory to practice .... The New American College, as a connect-

ed institution, would be committed to improving, in a very intentional way, the human condition.

Calling for the creation of the New American College is one thing, but creating it is something else entirely. To put it mildly, it is very hard to do. Since World War I, a strong tradition has developed that separates scholarly research from the goal of improving the human condition in the here and now. Disconnection from, rather then connection to, society became the operational style of the vast majority of America's colleges and universities (see Harkavy & Puckett 1991).

After 1945, higher education did connect. It connected, however, to distant, not local, problems. The Cold War became the defining issue that led to the development of the vast American "university system." Propelled by fear of and competition with the Soviet Union, American politicians, with significant support from the American public, unquestionably accepted requests from the "military-industrial-academic complex" for increased aid and support to higher education (Leslie 1993). Preoccupation with the Cold War did little to bridge the fragmentation of mission that already separated service from research and teaching, making effective engagement with the surrounding community all the more difficult (Harkavy & Puckett 1991; Harkavy 1992).

Tradition and fragmentation are certainly significant barriers to creating connected institutions. An additional barrier, however, may be even more formidable. There is a fundamental contradiction in the structure of the American research university itself, a contradiction that was built into its very creation. Daniel Coit Gilman, the founder of Johns Hopkins and central architect of the nineteenth century research university, claimed that one of his proudest accomplishments was "a school of science grafted on one of the oldest and most conservative classical colleges." (Gilman 1898). Although referring specifically to the merger of the Sheffield Scientific School with Yale College, Gilman felt that this achievement exemplified his contribution to American higher education.

As a product of a merger of the research university and the American college, the American research university was bound to develop severe tensions and contradictions from the joining of two markedly different entities. The research university was dedicated to specialized scholarship and service through specialized inquiry and studies. The American college, on the other hand, focused on general education, character building, and civic education. The college provided service to society through educating young people with, to use Benjamin Franklin's phrase, "an Inclination join'd with an Ability to serve." (Smith 1907). The research university has, of course, dominated this merger, creating an ethos and culture that rewards specialized study rather than the education of the next generation for moral, civic, and intellectual leadership.

CAN SERVICE LEARNING PROGRAMS CREATE CONNECTED INSTITUTIONS?

In the context of nearly 100 years of neglect, we are skeptical that service learning as it has evolved is adequate to a renewed agenda of civic education. Our position springs from trying to answer the question: What is the goal of the "service learning movement?" This is not merely an academic (in the pejorative sense) question. "It is," as Francis Bacon stated in 1620, "not possible to run a course aright when the goal itself is not rightly placed." In our judgment, the service learning movement has not "rightly placed" the goal. It has largely been concerned with advancing the civic consciousness and moral character of college students, arguing that service learning pedagogy also results in improved teaching and learning (e.g., Markus et al. 1993). Although service to the community is obviously an important component of service learning, it does not focus on solving core community problems.

The most influential work advocating, what might be termed, a "trickle down theory" of the impacts of service learning is Benjamin R. Barber's *An Aristocracy of Everyone: The Politics of Education and the Future of America* (1992). In a discussion of mandatory citizen education and community service, Barber asserts:

> To make people serve others may produce desirable behavior, but it does not create responsible and autonomous individuals. To make people participate in educational curricula that can empower them does create such individuals. *The ultimate goal is not to serve others but to learn to be free, which entails being responsible to others* [emphasis added]. (250-251)

According to this view, creating responsible and free persons is the ultimate objective of education. Solving core community problems is only a secondary outcome. However, the danger from adopting this perspective is that it may encourage the furtherance of service learning as a pedagogical equivalent of "exploitative" community-based research. Academics have often studied and written about poor, particularly minority, communities. The residents of those communities have largely been objects of study, sources of information for dissertations and articles that someday, somehow would contribute to making things better. Nevertheless, the problems of the poor remain with us, with not nearly enough notable examples of successful intervention attributable to the efforts of our vast research and educational resources.

Similarly, advocates and practitioners of service learning have tended to agree that the goal of that pedagogy is to educate college students for citizenship. Citizenship is learned by linking classroom experience to a service experience that is at best seen as doing "some" good for the community. The danger, however, is that the real beneficiaries are the deliverers, not the recipients, of the service. Someday, somehow, we are to imagine when we have effectively educated a critical mass of the "best and the brightest" for citizenship, things will be made better. Meanwhile, the causes of our societal problems have remained untouched, the distance between the haves and have nots has widened, and institutions of higher education have continued to engage in symbolic actions rather than producing knowledge for (to use Bacon's phrase) the "relief of man's estate."

Colleges and universities are in a unique position to "rightly place the goal" and "run [the]... course aright" by going beyond service learning (and its inherent limitations) to "strategic academically based community scholarship and service," which has as its primary goal contributing to the well-being of people in the community both in the here and now and in the future. It is service that is intrinsically tied to teaching and research and that aims to bring about *structural* community improvement (e.g., effective public schools, neighborhood economic development, strong community organizations) rather than simply to alleviate individual misery (e.g., feeding the hungry, sheltering the homeless, tutoring the "slow learner").

Strategic academically based community scholarship and service requires a comprehensive institutional response that engages the broad range of resources of the modern college and university (including the talents, abilities, and energy of undergraduates involved in traditional service and service learning activities) to solve the strategic problems of our time, including problems of health and disease (such as HIV infection).

Service learning, as we have argued, is much too weak a reed to get colleges and universities from here (internally-directed, self-referential institutions) to there (problem-solving, civic institutions). To mix metaphors, we need a stronger reed that can serve as a powerful lever for moving higher education and society forward. Even if we agree that strategic academically based community scholarship and service is the reed/lever, the question remains where and how do we apply it? Too general an approach, quite simply, will only take us so far. More concretely, what steps can colleges and universities take to transform their curricula and contribute to revitalizing American communities? An approach we have found helpful is to build on John Dewey's theory of instrumental intelligence and his identification of the core problem affecting modern society.

STRATEGIC ACADEMICALLY BASED COMMUNITY SCHOLARSHIP AND SERVICE AS A DEWEYAN APPROACH TO UNIVERSITY AND COMMUNITY REVITALIZATION

According to Dewey, genuine learning only occurs when human beings focus their attention, energies, and abilities on solving genuine "dilemmas" and "perplexities." Other mental "activity" fails to produce reflection and intellectual progress. As John W. Smith (1993) has written about Dewey's theory of instrumental intelligence: "Reflective thought is an active response to the challenge of the environment." In 1910, Dewey (1990) spelled out the basis of his real-world, problem-driven, problem-solving theory of instrumental intelligence as follows:

> Thinking begins in what may fairly be called a *forked-road* situation, a situation which is ambiguous, which presents a dilemma, which proposes alternatives. As long as our activity slides smoothly along from one thing to another, or as long as we permit our imagination to entertain fancies at pleasure, there is no call for reflection. Difficulty or obstruction in the way of reaching a belief brings us, however, to a pause ... *Demand for the solution of a perplexity is the steadying and guiding factor in the entire process of reflection* ... a question to be answered, an ambiguity to be resolved, sets up an end and holds the current of ideas to a definite channel ... [emphasis added].

> [In summary] ... the origin of thinking is some perplexity, confusion, or doubt: Thinking is not a case of spontaneous combustion; it does not occur just on "general principles." There is something specific which occasions and involves it. (ii)

Employing Dewey's theory of instrumental intelligence is, of course, only a starting point. There are an infinite number of perplexities and dilemmas for colleges and universities to focus upon. Which problem or set of problems are significant, basic, and strategic enough to lead to societal as well as intellectual progress? In 1927, in *The Public and Its Problems*, Dewey unequivocally identified the existence of "neighborly community" as indispensable for a well-functioning democratic society:

> There is no substitute for the vitality and depth of close and direct intercourse and attachment .... Democracy must begin at home, and its home is the neighborly community (213).

Dewey also noted that creating a genuinely democratic community is "in the first instance an intellectual problem" (147). Seven decades later, we still do not know how to create democratic neighborly communities. Events in Bosnia, the states of the former Soviet Union, South Africa, France, Germany, and Northern Ireland indicate that this very practical and core theoretical problem of the social sciences is more than an American dilemma. The problem of *how* to create these communities is a strategic problem of our time. As such, it is the problem most likely to advance the university's primary mission of advancing and transmitting knowledge to advance human welfare.

The particular strategic real world and intellectual problem many universities face is how to overcome the deep, pervasive, interrelated problems of their local environments. This concrete, immediate, practical and theoretical problem, needless to say, requires creative interdisciplinary interaction as well as cooperation with surrounding communities. Colleges and universities encompass the range of expertise needed to solve the complex, comprehensive, and interconnected problems found in our communities. To actually solve these problems, however, will require colleges and universities to change and increasingly become organizations that encourage and foster a Deweyan approach of "learning by strategic community problem-solving and real-world reflective doing."

CAN HIV/AIDS PREVENTION SERVE AS A CORE PROBLEM FOR STRATEGIC ACADEMICALLY BASED SCHOLARSHIP AND SERVICE LEARNING?

We believe that the challenges posed by the HIV/AIDS epidemic represent significant problems for most communities and that the social, economic, medical and ethical issues raised by the epidemic require the concerted attention of no less than the diverse resources represented in the modern college and university. The epidemic qualifies as a "forked-road situation" that involves numerous dilemmas and ambiguities with no easy solution. Although the infection still has no cure and preventive vaccines are yet to be found, transmission of the infection can be prevented. Nevertheless, nearly all preventive measures involve ethical and logistic dilemmas that have defied satisfactory resolution.

A brief overview of the major dilemmas created by attempts to prevent HIV infection and its progression to AIDS illustrates the magnitude of the problems our communities face. The most common routes of infection either involve unlawful behavior (e.g., use of needles to inject drugs) or private sexual acts, neither of which can be discussed beyond narrowly constraining moral boundaries. It is not surprising therefore that the stigma associated with the infection inhibits open identification of infected persons and makes testing a sensitive matter. Those who do identify themselves face unwarranted fears of HIV-infected persons, making accommodation to them in schools and workplaces difficult issues. Nevertheless, HIV-infected persons can go on living without any distinguishing signs for years, increasing the risks to themselves and others. Finally, the costs and difficulties of treatment are beyond the means of many of the afflicted, leaving them in dire need of assistance and care, a situation that strains the resources of our already inequitable medical systems. These dilemmas make the epidemic particularly problematic not only to our surrounding communities but also to undergraduates and their campus communities.

The risk of HIV infection for adolescents and young adults is particularly troubling. Among sexually active persons, adolescents and young adults have the highest rates of sexually transmitted disease, a situation that increases the risk to themselves and to campus communities (DiClemente 1992). In view of these risks, there remains a need to encourage students to take effective preventive action. However, the many social and moral conflicts associated with the infection inhibit open discussion of preventive action and reduce consistency in young people's adherence to prevention recommendations (Romer & Hornik 1992).

In recent years, the epidemic in the United States has moved primarily from afflicting gay men to now threatening residents of poor non-white communities, including women and their children (CDC 1996a,b). The needs of these constituencies are especially prone to neglect, making the infection even more likely to spread in their communities. Recent advances make it possible to prevent the infection in newborns, but issues of testing and confidentiality create ethical and medical conflicts that have no simple solution. These conflicts become even more problematic when poor women who are dependent on publicly-financed health care must suffer the effects of government imposed testing.

As with most real-world problems, most solutions raise moral as well financial dilemmas. It is no surprise therefore that a multitude of disciplines can provide context and methodologies for helping to resolve the contradictions of the epidemic. In all likelihood, true resolution will require the integration of disciplines. Public health and epidemiology are only the most basic sources of insight into the problem. For example, legal and public policy studies are critical for understanding the role of the criminal justice system in banning the use of needles and drugs, policies that may only encourage the underground use of these products. Political science is helpful for probing the barriers that prevent informed discussion of the epidemic and that inhibit government action to establish effective prevention programs. The sociology of poverty is helpful in understanding why impoverished communities now bear the brunt of the epidemic. The history of medicine can explore past failures to cope with sexually-transmitted diseases and other stigmatizing illnesses. Cultural anthropology can provide insight into the reasons why behavior that is risky can become normative in certain groups and impervious to public-health warnings and control. Gender studies can help to understand the stigma associated with gay victims of the disease and the conflicts produced by prevention that is dependent on male behavior (i.e., condom use). And the list goes on.

Despite the wealth of inter-disciplinary insight that has been created in recent years, there are no simple or universally accepted solutions to controlling the epidemic or to reducing the suffering it creates. Direct experience in confronting the epidemic will not only reinforce this conclusion but also challenge faculty and students to seek solutions that existing scholarship has yet to recognize. This is all the more reason for encouraging direct involvement in service. Such service can range from providing HIV/AIDS-prevention education to adolescents (including fellow undergraduates) and other community members, helping to staff AIDS hotlines, assisting food banks that serve AIDS patients, counselling persons affected by the disease, and advocating for greater understanding of the epidemic in the community.

However, our concerns about the structure of service learning and its role within the academy alert us to the need to encourage strategic partnerships in designing academically based HIV/AIDS prevention programs. By engaging the epidemic in the community, students and faculty can appreciate at first hand the conflicts and obstacles posed by the disease and the difficult challenges that coping with these issues pose. Providing solutions to the problems will require research and thoughtful engagement by faculty, students, and community partners working together to overcome the obstacles that the epidemic creates. Finally, whatever solutions are suggested will require action on the part of both campus and community partners to see if the solutions are effective. In short, we envision a process of partnership, research, reflection, and action. Clearly, creating partnerships with community organizations is a critical first step in advancing this agenda, as we discuss in the next section.

CREATING PARTNERSHIPS IN A STRATEGIC APPROACH TO HIV/AIDS PREVENTION

If service learning is to be harnessed as a vehicle for strategic community problem solving, then our experience suggests that partnerships with existing community organizations are critical. There are several reasons for focusing on these partnerships. First, community organizations are the most likely to be able to provide the experience and expertise needed to develop good strategies for intervention in the community. Their role as service providers places them at the forefront of the problem. Second, community organizations are most likely to need the kind of immediate and long-term assistance that a service-learning effort can provide. In return for this assistance, they can help to supervise students placed in their charge. Third, community organizations are most likely to be in the position to implement whatever strategic goals are identified as solutions to community problems.

In our development of service learning at the University of Pennsylvania, we have created linkages with several local public schools that are interested in collaborating with our students and faculty to improve their education programs and the health and welfare of their communities (see Harkavy & Puckett 1991; Sommerfeld 1996). An ongoing replication of the program at the University of Alabama at Birmingham has focused directly on HIV/AIDS education and prevention in local schools. Similar partnerships will be beneficial in creating programs to cope with the HIV epidemic. We describe four programs in very different settings that have begun the process of partnership development. As would be expected, programs are still in the early stages of developing strategic relationships with community partners. The ones we describe vary in their development but are illustrative of the many ways in which service can be strategically directed to resolving community problems. In addition, the examples provide some indication of what can be realistically achieved in the early stages of program development.

Gannon University: The recent work of one university we have studied as part of a statewide evaluation of an AmeriCorps service-learning program in Pennsylvania (Romer & Harkavy 1996) is an example of a partnership in a rural setting where HIV/AIDS education and awareness building are priority issues. Gannon University, in rural Erie county, has devoted considerable effort toward developing campus-wide service-learning programs related to HIV/AIDS prevention. Their programs involve students as part-time AmeriCorps members in a host of activities on both the campus and in the surrounding rural area. Partnerships have been established with both the county health department and with local organizations that receive prevention-services funding from CDC. Students also work with health educators on campus to coordinate HIV/AIDS week, to staff a campus AIDS Action Team, and to recruit volunteers for service in community HIV/AIDS prevention.

The activities that students engage in cover the entire range described earlier, and there is considerable evidence from student reports that the experience is unique and unattainable through classroom-based pedagogy alone. For our purposes, however, we wish to emphasize the important role that liaisons with both campus and community organizations play in the service-learning effort. Community partners define the services that students can provide, and they value the assistance that the students offer. At the same time, students recognize the difficulties inherent in the services the organizations provide. Establishing these connections has been an important accomplishment in the Gannon program. As their service-learning program matures, these connections will allow the development of serious intellectual interchange between the faculty, students and service organizations that can lead to a more strategic focus for future service learning activities.

University of Alabama at Birmingham: Another program recently started at UAB is an example of how partnerships can be created between a large urban research university and its neighboring community. As a result of funding to create partnerships with local schools, UAB is coordinating a range of programs that the local schools have identified as high priorities for intervention by the University. One such priority is assistance in the development of HIV/AIDS education for a middle school in a neighborhood that is experiencing increasing rates of HIV infection but that has not had much personal experience with the epidemic. As a result, the school is concerned that the youth will need help to understand the risks and unjustified fears associated with the infection.

In response to this need, the School of Public Health at UAB has brought its experts in HIV/AIDS education together to develop a program to train students in the school as peer educators. This program follows an earlier effort in the partnership to educate students as peer leaders in violence reduction and conflict resolution. The success of that effort suggested that a similar program could be initiated for HIV/AIDS education. Although it is too early to see the effects of this plan, it is anticipated that undergraduates will become involved in the training program as part of their health education courses at the School of Education. The School of Social Work may also play a role in directing the program (Struzick 1996).

In both of these examples, the programs are in the early stages of development. The focus has been on creating interventions in the community that exploit the knowledge and abilities of undergraduates and faculty. At the same time, they are directed toward the problems that community organizations have identified as critical to their mission. Future development of these programs will benefit from ongoing participation of students in courses designed to engage in real-world problem solving concerning HIV infection in local communities. Questions that will undoubtedly arise as the programs mature will include finding better ways to educate communities that are resistant to the risk of HIV and that are insufficiently sensitive to the suffering that the epidemic has inflicted. Included in this challenge is the undergraduate community itself. In addition, issues of adequate medical care in both rural and urban areas, as well as the problems associated with the stigma of testing, will also arise. As these issues are debated by students and faculty, a dialogue can develop between the campus and its partners that can allow both sides to define ways in which new strategies for coping with the epidemic can be tested by their partnership. This is the potential that a campus-wide program can achieve.

San Francisco State University: A maturing program at SFSU illustrates how service-learning can progress through collaboration across campuses in an urban AIDS epicenter. The City of Service program at the University links students from its own as well as three other campuses (University of California at San Francisco, City College of San Francisco, and New College of California) with local agencies, including those that provide HIV/AIDS services and prevention. With funding from the Learn and Serve Program of the National Center for Community Service, City of Service finds agencies in the city that can use the assistance of undergraduates and arranges placements for students from all four campuses. Students and faculty from service-learning courses also use the program to identify appropriate agencies for their own placement needs.

Dr. Felix Kury of San Francisco State teaches a service-learning course, titled "Latino Health Care Perspectives," that has sent students to the program for several years. Students are required to spend 30 hours during the semester in their community placement. In these placements, students engage in a variety of activities, such as assisting in programming for residential AIDS patients and educating Latino and African-American high school students. Students use their experiences from these activities in class when discussing their required readings and write a paper that relates the experience to course content. The community partners benefit from having Latino and African-American students assist them in their work.

Another interesting partnership in the College of Health Services at San Francisco State enrolls students working toward a degree in nutrition science. Students from this class devote 30 hours of service to a residence center for AIDS patients where finding appetizing and health-preserving meals is a challenge. As part of their service, students work with the food preparation staff to create menus that are nutritionally appropriate for the residents, an activity that uses their expertise in creative ways.

City of Service staff maintain contact with partner agencies throughout the semester and conduct follow-up evaluations to determine if their needs are being met. In this process, the needs of both the campus and the community can be monitored so that the program serves both sides of the partnership.

Bryn Mawr College: An example of a more highly developed strategic service-learning class directed toward HIV/AIDS has been in existence since 1990 at Bryn Mawr College, in suburban Philadelphia. Dr. Judith Porter, a professor in the sociology department, is an active researcher in the HIV/AIDS-prevention field who has created a service learning seminar for advanced undergraduates that not only provides a rigorous overview of the field but also exposes students to the realities of HIV/AIDS prevention in poor Latino and Black neighborhoods of Philadelphia (Porter & Schwartz

1993). Students spend four hours a week serving in one of four agencies that provide prevention services such as needle exchange for injecting drug users. The experiences gained in those settings provide a grounding in the epidemic that far exceeds what is available in readings. Indeed, staff in the community sites visit the classroom to discuss issues of prevention and treatment with students.

Dr. Porter reports to us that the course is a clear success. Students learn. They find their lives changed by the experience. Many pursue careers in public health and medicine as a result. However, the critical component in the course's success is the strong relationship that Dr. Porter maintains with the sites where her students volunteer. She also works in the same settings and conducts research on projects related to their activities. This liaison allows Dr. Porter not only to monitor her students' activities but also to be sensitive to the same experiences they encounter. As a result of the strong connection with the community sites, students not only complete a challenging syllabus but also suggest solutions to problems that the agencies face. Some create newsletters for clients to help disseminate prevention information. Others have created brochures on such topics as nutrition for HIV-infected persons. Papers written by students on their service experience are made available to the agencies, often with interesting suggestions about their services.

MOVING TOWARD IMPLEMENTATION

The examples we provide are only a few of the many programs that have been created to forge links between undergraduate education and HIV/AIDS prevention in the community. Nevertheless, these examples span a range of campuses and local communities. It is clear from these examples that the particular partnerships that arise will depend on the relationships that faculty and staff have with local organizations and schools. Faculty strengths and interests will undoubtedly play a large role in the selection of sites and the types of interventions selected. However, as the examples at several campuses illustrate, central coordination of service learning encourages community organizations to seek help from the campus and stimulates the identification of service-learning opportunities for faculty and students.

Faculty who wish to embark on the journey of establishing partnerships in strategic academically based service learning are likely to find the rewards quite substantial. Faculty members at the University of Pennsylvania who had taught courses for many years without a service component find the new experience truly energizing. However, it must also be emphasized that adopting a problem-solving orientation directed to the community requires a different relationship between faculty and students from the traditional roles typically adopted. In the context of real-world problem solving, faculty and students are collaborators trying to understand the problems in the community. Although faculty have far more expertise in their discipline, the experiences that students gain from their service are as valuable to faculty understanding as to the students themselves. Experiences in the community become primary material for critiquing theory and placing existing scholarship in context. Some faculty find journal writing, in-class discussion, and paper assignments that focus on service experiences helpful in promoting the goals of service learning. As Dr. Porter's course suggests, community representatives can play a valuable role in the classroom by leading discussion and sharing their experiences.

Sending students off campus also has its risks. Students engaged in HIV/AIDS prevention may venture into crime-ridden neighborhoods or expose themselves to emotionally challenging experiences. These concerns can be anticipated by encouraging prudent travel and behavior in risky settings, and by providing opportunities for counselling and discussion for those requiring such assistance. In some cases, students are asked to sign contracts that acknowledge the risks and the responsibilities that they and their faculty members assume. Such contracts may also reveal risks that infected persons can suffer (e.g., patronizing attitudes or exposure to additional infections) and ways to avoid these outcomes.

Materials that have already been tested in community settings can provide some guidance for the uninitiated in the field of HIV/AIDS prevention. Numerous education guides have been created for use by undergraduates in reaching out to local schools and other community organizations. For example, the American Student Medical Association has developed a program for medical students that has been adapted for use by undergraduates (Karabelnik & Gold 1994). The critical component is faculty interest and partnerships with community (and campus) service sites.

All this noted, however, the emphasis on community-campus partnerships to solve problems of the community is still relatively new. Models of effective implementation are still being created and refined. As this work progresses, the need for sharing the successes and failures of these efforts will increase so that programs in similar circumstances can benefit from the experience and use it to develop and refine their own programs.

ISSUES OF EVALUATION

As programs evolve, a critical question that will arise is whether the campus-community partnership has succeeded in its goals. This is a multi-faceted issue. Some of the goals focus on student achievement and satisfaction with service-learning courses.

Do students find the experience challenging and worthwhile? Do the courses draw students? Do students learn? Research on the effects of service-learning is still in its infancy. However, what evidence there is suggests that service-learning courses can be as rigorous as traditional courses. Indeed, more course content may be mastered by students in service-learning classes than in traditional lecture and discussion-based classes, and students may find the experience more stimulating (e.g., Markus et al. 1993).

A more difficult issue revolves around assessing the impact of service-based learning on the solution of community and campus problems. Here evaluations will be needed that assess educational and other objectives on an ongoing basis in the community sites where service activities are directed. Truly strategic service learning will incorporate evaluation as part of the educational program because it is only through feedback to the partnership that progress can be assessed. At a minimum, community partners should be asked to gauge their assessment of the collaboration and areas for continued development. In addition, research to assess progress toward program goals will also be desirable. For example, if a public school is a site for HIV/AIDS prevention outreach, then surveys on an ongoing basis will be conducted with the students to see if HIV/AIDS education objectives are being reached (e.g., knowledge of risk behaviors, appropriate understanding of false risks of infection, and relevant steps for prevention, etc.). Other objectives, such as greater respect for sexual partners or civic awareness about the effects of communicable diseases, might also be a focus. Such surveys could be a responsibility of undergraduates in other courses (e.g., introductory research design) and serve as a learning tool in themselves.

HOW TO GET STARTED

HIV/AIDS prevention could be a valuable focus for undergraduate curricula and for strategic academically based service learning. HIV infection is a serious problem for communities that poses dilemmas for every solution that has been offered. Furthermore, the health and welfare of youth both on the campus and in the wider community is a concern that our colleges and universities should not ignore. The study of the epidemic as it affects both the campus and the surrounding community and methods of coping with it can be educationally rewarding as well as supportive of the goals of the engaged academy outlined so eloquently by Boyer (1994).

To conclude, we suggest the following first steps to those who wish to take a leadership role on their campus:

1. Identify potentially interested faculty to discuss the development of service learning courses with an HIV/AIDS focus.

2. Identify and create links with appropriate community and campus partners concerned with HIV/AIDS prevention and treatment.

3. If needed, explore funding sources to support your campus service learning efforts. One such effort might be to create a campus-wide clearing-house to encourage both the surrounding community and the campus to identify service learning opportunities.

4. Connect other faculty with interests in service learning to the HIV/AIDS effort.

5. Begin to create an integrated service learning agenda for the campus through seminars, speakers, discussion groups, and campus media.

References for this essay may be found on page 147.

RESOURCES FOR FURTHER DISCUSSION OF SERVICE LEARNING

We recommend the following sources for further discussion of recent developments in the service learning movement.

Service Learning in Higher Education: Concepts and Practices, edited by Barbara Jacoby. San Francisco: Jossey-Bass, 1997.

University-Community Collaborations for the Twenty-First Century: Outreach Scholarship for Youth and Families, edited by Richard M. Lerner and Lou Anna K. Simon. Garland Publishing, 1998.

Successful Service Learning Programs, by Ed Zlotkowski. Boulton, MA: Anchor Books, 1998.

"Service Learning." A special issue of *Metropolitan Universities*, vol. 7(l), 1996.

Combining Service and Learning, edited by J. Kendall. Raleigh, NC: National Society for Experiential Education, 1990.

Where's the Learning in Service Learning, edited by Janet Eyler and Dwight Giles, San Francisco: Jossey Bass, 1999.

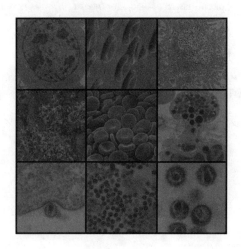

SIX

Learning About AIDS and Ethics in a Liberal Democracy

Nora Kizer Bell

Wesleyan College

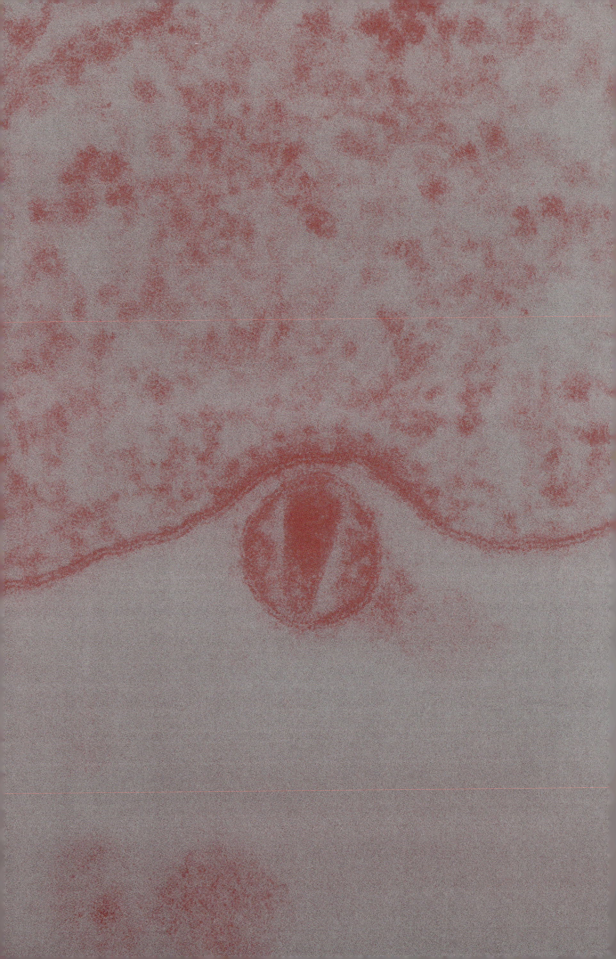

As a part of their desire to help students acquire the benefits of a liberal arts education, many educational leaders have begun to focus attention on ethics as integral to liberal learning. Recalling a time when imparting notions of citizenship, community service, and community values were important goals in most educational contexts, these educators believe that their mission includes helping students learn to be both good persons and good citizens. As a consequence, educational leaders are seeking ways to help students understand the moral implications of their beliefs and actions; they are searching for strategies that will help them teach reflective moral judgment. Increasingly, those of us in higher education hope to educate what Martha Nussbaum calls the Diogenesian "world citizen"—a human being capable not only of learning the facts but capable as well of love and concern, a citizen who is both empathetic and skilled in the ways of critical analysis and logic (Prashad 1999).

With similar urgency, educational leaders are demonstrating an awareness that ethical reasoning and capacity are important forms of learning and ways of thinking and doing that are critical to a broad range of professional education and eventual professional practice. Accordingly, over the past two decades there has been a new emphasis on ethics in professional programs like law, medicine, nursing, business, teacher preparation, communications, journalism/mass media, and others. This attention to ethics and moral reasoning in professional practice seeks to inculcate a voluntary interest in and disposition toward ethical action.

And, of course, educators are cognizant of the place that choices with ethical content have in the lives of students within their campuses and neighboring communities. Students are moral actors and moral agents, and they continually confront questions that require a higher level of moral deliberation. Higher education leaders see a need to help students and others address, for example, issues of bigotry and prejudice, date rape, binge drinking, academic dishonesty, abusive relationships—all issues where students' choices have significant moral ramifications.

Hence, higher education leaders, among others, search for ways to refresh and strengthen the teaching of ethics. And as they do, it has been common to explore a variety of ways ethics might be "taught"—from exploring the great traditions in ethical thinking, such as utilitarianism, deontology, relativism, orthodoxy, pragmatism, and feminism, to using tough issues, like the death penalty or abortion, to analyzing case studies and arguments.

Into this mix comes HIV/AIDS—literally a Pandora's box of traditional ethical dilemmas interspersed with some new ones that demand careful consideration. The issues and dilemmas generated by HIV/AIDS are familiar to those of us who have long worried about HIV/AIDS—and they are sharply contested, hotly debated public matters, such as:

- partner notification
- needle exchange
- right to treatment
- right to refuse treatment
- allocation of scarce resources
- justice and desert
- right to information
- right to be free from offensive, unsolicited information

- liberty versus control
- "duty to care"
- innocence
- individual responsibility
- public versus private freedom
- prejudice
- self-worth
- informed consent

The issues raised by HIV/AIDS, although not new, continue to be among the most challenging of our times—both medically and socially. While AIDS has been the subject of public debate and controversy since it was first discovered in the early 1980s, much of the conversation and discussion of AIDS has been rhetorical and aimed at provocation. It has often been less than thoughtful or analytical. As a result, the ethical and policy dimensions of HIV disease have been particularly complicated to address.

But, these issues are *not* philosophical abstractions. They represent real world dilemmas that come into play daily in the interactions of students with one another, in the considerations of authority figures on campuses and those for whom they are responsible, and in the determinations of policy makers. An examination of the ethical issues raised by HIV disease—particularly the ethical issues in AIDS education—thus seems a natural forum for developing ethical reasoning and heightening moral sensitivities.

In past iterations, for the most part, AIDS and HIV were the domain of public health officials, epidemiologists, virologists, immunologists, and physicians and others who dealt with sexually transmitted diseases. AIDS was hardly the subject matter of the traditional liberal educational curriculum. In fact, some might ask what liberal inquiry could possibly bring to bear on the questions raised by AIDS and HIV disease. Apart from the intellectual development that might occur if HIV disease is the subject matter around which ethical deliberation is learned, what recommends HIV disease as a topic peculiarly suited to study in the academy?

One obvious answer might be that HIV disease is a serious public and practical issue that requires for its solution the talents and minds of students and faculty engaged in the pursuit of higher education. Certainly, the issues raised by AIDS and HIV cover a very broad range of topics that need to be covered in any good undergraduate learning experience that attempts to teach ethics, civic engagement, and personal agency or responsibility.

And there are a number of questions that one might hope would be answered by a study of HIV disease: Will such study help affect individual behavior? In what ways? Will it positively influence individual civic engagement? Will this help meet campus goals of health promotion and disease prevention? Will it carry any particular "imperatives"? What could those imperatives be? Will it teach an understanding of differing points of view? Will it validate or frustrate relativism?

Let me suggest a different reason to pursue the study of HIV/AIDS in the context of liberal education—one that takes us beyond the expectation that the liberal arts should be intertwined with current, real world issues and one that takes us beyond a view of HIV/AIDS that speaks only to health promotion or traditional models of student wellness. The study of HIV/AIDS as a part of one's training in the liberal arts speaks uniquely to the integrity of the educational experience itself. In other words, if we accept democratic ideals as one of the conceptual cornerstones of American higher education, there are significant implications in that for how we conceive both AIDS education and liberal education.

HIV AND THE INTEGRITY OF THE EDUCATIONAL EXPERIENCE

Many ethical issues in AIDS education arise because we take the notion of democratic education very seriously. The moral debate over appropriate forms of AIDS education has produced no clear consensus on how early education should begin, to which groups it should be directed, who should do it, how long it should be continued, what kinds of information it should include, and whether coercion or compulsion will be more effective in achieving public health educational goals. And, in a liberal democracy, we do not easily entertain a conception of education that has complete mind or behavior control as its mission.

Unfortunately, there has been no clear statement of what moral principles might motivate one to choose education as against choosing compulsion. And there is still heated debate over how effective educational programs have been to date in accomplishing public health objectives. In short, a great many issues in AIDS education call for careful examination.

Consider, for example, the goals of AIDS education since the 1980s. The standard for success in AIDS education has seemed clear—to effect behavior change. Furthermore, it has seemed equally clear that the bottom line for those in AIDS prevention, the public health goal in much of AIDS education, has been the elimination of disease—zero transmission, 100 percent risk reduction. Short of that, public health efforts are said to have failed. Neither the critics nor the proponents of most AIDS educational efforts distinguished the educational goal of dispensing information to persons likely to be infected/affected from the goal of restructuring the behaviors of those persons.

DEMOCRATIC EDUCATION AND FREEDOM

By its very nature, democratic education—that is, education that occurs in the context of a liberal democracy—will eventuate in something less than complete compliance with, or complete assimilation to, its instructional mission. A truly democratic society is willing to give up some degree of control of citizens' behavior in order to encourage the responsible exercise of individual freedom. A commitment to democratic education means, therefore, accepting compromise in its results. This is especially true in a culture that is pluralistic (Gutmann 1987).

AIDS education understood in such a context—and, hence, education itself—must accommodate all kinds of cultural perspectives and individual variations, handicaps, strengths, and proclivities. Surely, part of what it means to accept the concept of democratic education is to accept that education should not advance any particular cultural perspective any more than education can solve the myriad of problems confronting those whom it seeks to educate. And, of course, AIDS is only one of a number of social problems for which this claim has relevance. Rather than recommend draconian measures of behavior control, the concept of democratic education seems to suggest offering people information about a range of options, all of which can have better or worse impact on their lives. It also seems to commit us to offering various perspectives as lenses through which to understand the various dimensions of HIV disease. Such a conception of education relies heavily on the conviction that not everyone will be attracted to the same options and that, even if they are, they will be able to achieve them to greater or lesser degrees. Furthermore, such a conception of education underscores the value of informed, yet voluntary choice.

Thus, even if we were to agree that completely eliminating risky behaviors is desirable in combating the spread of HIV and should be advocated in AIDS education programs, our commitment to the desirability of democratic education ensures that AIDS education programs may not accomplish that end.

If AIDS education cannot accomplish eliminating behaviors that transmit HIV—

and if education in general cannot guarantee outcomes among its students—what is there about the concept of democratic education to recommend it? Here we must evaluate what should count as criteria for success in education.

For a democratic society that places a high value on pluralism, the principle of respect for persons has important moral force. Respecting persons requires a presumption in favor of individual responsibility. The principle of respect for persons requires not only that we accept all persons as equally possessing moral status and moral agency, but also that we treat them with such respect, that we affirm their moral right to be treated equitably, and that we affirm their moral right to be different. The principle of respect for persons also requires that we provide persons with the tools and information essential for exercising their moral agency. Ensuring respect for persons is accomplished, to use Gutmann's language, by the principles of nonrepression and nondiscrimination (Gutmann 1987). The authority of democratic education must be constrained to accomplish these ends.

The criteria for a successful AIDS education program in such a context might be vastly different from the way some public health educators conceive it. Under such a democratic conception, strategies for reducing transmission of HIV must rely heavily on moral persuasion, rational deliberation, and, hence, on the availability of current and accurate information on HIV transmission and prevention. Under such a conception of education, success is achieved if persons and societies are enabled to govern themselves. Success is achieved if persons can be participants in their own learning and if they can differentiate and accept responsibility for moral choices.

AIDS education has been successful if persons are enabled, for example, to establish norms of mutual protection and self-respect that would allow them to change behaviors and preserve their social identification. Proponents of such a conception of education have confidence that people will learn, albeit at different rates and in different ways. Their learning will be conditioned by their various perspectives. Measuring success under such a conception of education means something vastly different from quantifying outcomes or determining whether particular percentages of persons change their behaviors.

One of the principles that is said to provide the philosophical underpinnings for a liberal democracy derives from a principle articulated by John Stuart Mill and typically identified as the "harm principle": one is free to do as one chooses so long as those actions harm no one else. This principle, while often used to justify paternalistic interventions designed to prevent harm to others, does not justify limiting one's freedom for one's own good. A commitment to the concept of democratic education, then, suggests not only that we cannot eliminate all undesirable behaviors that threaten others in society, but also that it is inappropriate to seek to prevent voluntarily chosen self-destructive behavior. We can educate and inform; we can provide techniques and training; we can urge and persuade. We cannot force learning.

Such a conception of education obviously involves certain risks or liabilities—namely, that some people will learn but will not change their behaviors, that they will forget, that they will make mistakes—and, in the case of HIV/AIDS, that the disease will not be entirely eliminated. Education may even make some persons more willing to take risks with themselves and others than they were before—say, because they learn that the possibility of infection from HIV from one risky behavior is considerably smaller than they originally believed. Education could make persons less responsible in that sense than they were before. But, of course, these are all risks inherent in an educational enterprise understood as democratic.

For many participating in policy decisions, the undesirability of such risks has led to suggestions that society pursue HIV/AIDS prevention alternatives other than education. And it is for precisely that reason that the study of HIV/AIDS seems most appropriate for those involved in liberal learning in the academy.

HIV EDUCATION AND LIBERAL EDUCATION

Whether one adopts the more traditional model of liberal education (as high culture, distinct from practical concerns) or the Deweyan model of liberal education (as the search for truth that connects theory with practice), surely we think of liberal education as integrated learning—integration to include character development along with intellectual development, practical knowledge combined with academic knowledge, an education that seeks to encourage enlightened citizenship. The perspective that a commitment to democratic education brings to the discussion of AIDS education is revealing of what liberal education's aims must be.

A liberal arts education offers the foundation to enrich capacities of judgment, discernment, curiosity, critical thinking, conscience and compassion—knowledge that avows the power and purpose of the human spirit. A liberal arts education—one committed to the principles of liberal democracy—provides the place where personal abilities can blossom; it opens the mind to opportunities to learn. It has an obligation to be honest, to meet the needs of those being taught, to engage them in learning, to encourage more learning, to connect with their inner spirit, to help its students continue to become—rather than seeking to produce a finished product.

As I indicated earlier in this essay, HIV/AIDS offers a unique perspective from which to think about the educational enterprise. HIV/AIDS provides an especially rich context against which to explore our shared morality, against which to develop a capacity for ethical reasoning. And AIDS educational efforts themselves are instructive of how to evaluate the aims of liberal education. It is one thing to try to determine whether we should have AIDS education and what that education should include. In a democratic society, there really is no choice whether or not to educate persons about a disease as potentially devastating as AIDS. We have a responsibility to provide that education, whether or not it eventuates in behavior change. The fact that we have a responsibility in a liberal democracy to provide AIDS education says nothing, however, about whether society should or should not appeal to punishment or coercion as strategies for containing HIV transmission.

Similarly, today's educational leaders would argue that we have a responsibility to ensure that our students learn to understand and appreciate the varieties of ethical thinking—whether or not they become "fully" ethical persons. In a democratic society, there really is no choice whether or not to provide students with an opportunity to develop this dimension of their thinking and reasoning. The issues involved in sorting out how to think about the consequences of failing to "get" the educational message should not, however, be conflated with whether we will or will not make appeal to coercive measures to ensure compliance with our instructional goal.

Only if we think that education must necessarily eventuate in specific behaviors are we pushed to think that we must choose between it and coercion. So, for example, while we might agree that HIV/AIDS education should include telling people what their responsibilities to others are and helping them learn how to fulfill those responsibilities and obligations they accept, it is a very different enterprise to determine what will happen to persons who fail to choose to heed that message. Unfortunately, one reason coercion or compulsion appeals to so many persons is that it provides an outlet for the anger and resentment felt toward those whose lifestyles or behaviors stand in stark contrast to the educational message. So, for example, the preference for compulsion seems to be correlated with the belief that persons who contract HIV/AIDS are deficient in moral character or self control—that they have chosen immoral behavior and are, therefore, morally culpable rather than victims (Reamer 1983).

Communicating information through education is easy; changing behaviors, especially risky behaviors, is not. If one adopts the eliminative or compliance approach, one is likely to opt merely for a strategy of compulsion or coercion. In a democratic society, however, it is the process that is as important as the result.

In the end, our common health "cannot be separated from a concern for democracy and its requirements for an educated electorate, for [our common] health in its broadest sense is [our common] welfare and its foundations lie in social justice" (Kreiger & Lashof 1988).

References for this essay may be found on page 149.

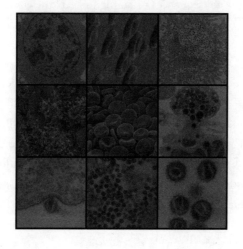

SEVEN

Placing HIV/AIDS in Perspective: A Question of History?

Robert E. Fullilove and
Mindy Thompson Fullilove, M.D.
Columbia University

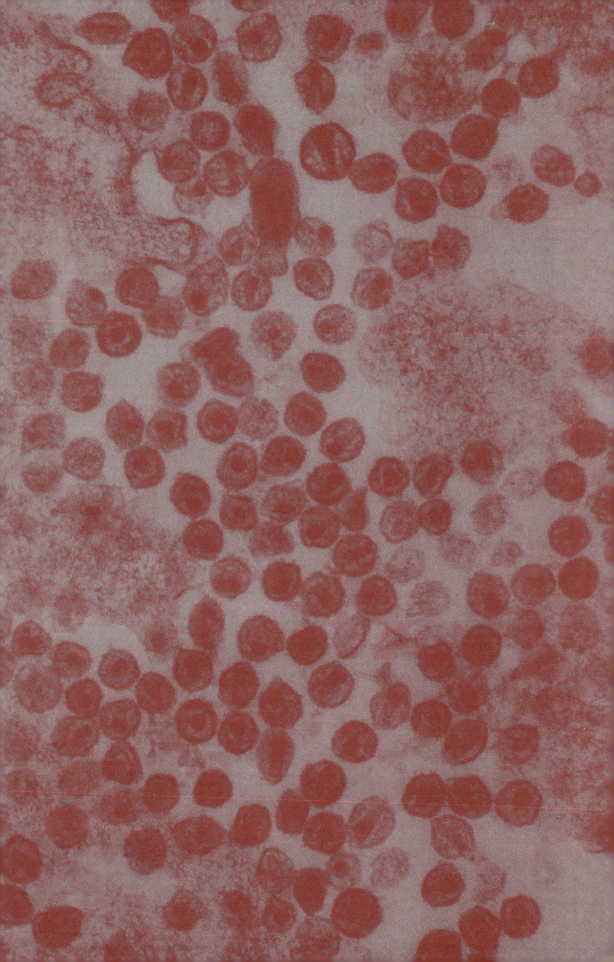

S talin said, "One death is a tragedy. A million deaths is a statistic." This essay
explores the relationship between the AIDS pandemic—now measured in the
millions—race, and the failure of the national dialogue about these topics. Our
opinions are those of two African American AIDS researchers who have been engaged
in the investigation of the epidemiology of HIV infection in poor communities of color
in the United States. We do not, therefore, approach this issue with the detachment
that scientists often claim is essential in the creation of an unbiased view of a socially
and politically charged subject such as AIDS.

However, we are also educators who have been privileged to involve dozens of students in our work and who have benefited tremendously from lively classroom debates
with them about the significance of our research, our findings, and our conclusions. In
the pages that follow we hope to present a synthesis of the issues that this series of
interactions and conversations have illuminated.

We begin with the premise that our efforts to inform and educate people about the
AIDS pandemic are significantly complicated by the ghosts of our national history.
HIV infection is, at once, a microscopic, personal, communal, national, and global
phenomenon.

Complicating efforts to mount an effective national campaign against the epidemic, however, is the fact that the complexion of HIV/AIDS is increasingly black and
brown. Since the mid-90s, the majority of new cases of AIDS in the United States
have been reported among African Americans and Latinos. The legacy of distrust that
haunts race relations in this country has now extended to the dialogue that members of
HIV-affected communities have with each other and with the government about the
epidemic and about the best strategies for combating it.

In subsequent sections of this essay, we will discuss this dialogue and show how it
is tinged with myths, rumors, and contemporary legends about the true origins of
HIV/AIDS and about the true nature of the government's interest in fighting the epidemic. Rather than dismiss folk beliefs about the epidemic as the product of ignorance
and a lack of sophistication about science and medicine, we wish to assert—following
the work of African American anthropologist Patricia Turner—that these beliefs provide an important glimpse into the larger dynamic of race relations in the United
States. There will be no progress in our efforts to defeat HIV/AIDS, we maintain,
until we recognize how much the epidemic is being fueled by unresolved national
debates about how to solve the problems of race.

HIV/AIDS: What Is It Really?

Jonathan Mann (1998) was fond of remarking that AIDS is a window on the world, a prism through which we are able to see all of the dilemmas, conflicts, and unresolved social issues of the 20th century. In an article written for *Scientific American* and published a few months before his untimely death, he wrote:

> Epidemiologists have been dismayed to uncover a societal level factor influencing the distribution [of AIDS in the world]: groups whose human rights are least respected are the most affected. As epidemics mature within communities and countries, the brunt of the epidemic often shifts from the primary population in which HIV first appeared to those who were socially marginalized or discriminated against before the epidemic began.

Mann's insistence that HIV/AIDS is first and foremost a human rights issue has been a dominant theme in our research and teaching. However, it has often been difficult to convince both our fellow researchers and our students that such a view is useful. We are often asked "Are you trying to say that until we cure poverty, discrimination, and racism, we'll be powerless to stop AIDS? Why not ask us to suspend the law of gravity as well?"

The more we have pondered the manner in which our message has been received, the more we have come to believe that our difficulties in making a convincing case are bound up, not surprisingly, in the national struggle to make sense of the true meaning of race, discrimination, and health in the United States. Moreover, the fact that we are African American researchers engaged in an on-going series of research efforts to understand this problem has been both a blessing and a curse.

The blessing has been that, in more than fifteen years of research on public health in communities of color, we have been granted access to many people and settings that are closed to white researchers. We have been privy to conversations that are closed to "outsiders" and have engaged in discussions about sex and drugs that have revealed the most intimate secrets of the communities where we have worked (see list of references).

The curse has been that our efforts to look beyond race to examine the critical role that poverty, racism, and geographic isolation play in centering the HIV/AIDS epidemic in crumbling, disintegrating ghettos (such as the South Bronx or Harlem in New York City, or the Central Ward of Newark, New Jersey) have often been treated as being "very interesting" but having no practical utility. Some examination of the issues we have confronted may prove useful.

AIDS AND RACE

In 1986, while the epidemic was comparatively young, we were asked to examine why AIDS cases were disproportionately represented among minority populations. In that year African Americans and Latinos comprised approximately 17 percent of the United States population but approximately 40 percent of the cumulative cases of AIDS reported to the United States Centers for Disease Control and Prevention (CDC) since 1981. (For current statistics, see the CDC Website at http://www.cdc.gov/scientific.htm.) The connection between AIDS and race was the subject of much speculation then, as now. Although we were new initiates to public health research, we were struck by the degree to which no one questioned the logic of having "race" serve as one of the primary "prisms"—to borrow from Jonathan Mann's metaphor—through which we would try to make sense of the epidemiology of HIV/AIDS.

Race, it should be recalled, is fundamentally an arbitrary classification scheme that is used to assign members of the human family to groups according to inherited physical traits such as skin color, hair texture, and so on. As a consequence, one might expect that race-based examinations of HIV/AIDS would be founded in the same kind of logic as research into the genetic relationships between, say, sickle cell disease and the black race.

The reality, of course, is far more complex. Gene science has little if any relevance for explaining the prevalence of HIV infection among people of color in the United States. Race in the context of the HIV/AIDS epidemic is a proxy for a host of social, economic, political, geographical, and cultural factors, all of which interact with an equally complicated array of factors that are associated with risk for HIV infection. Simply put, race is not the issue, racism is. In this context racism might be described as the set of social and political dynamics that will determine an individual's odds for succeeding or failing in life based largely, if not exclusively, on the individual's race.

While few scientists disagree with this formulation, race, not racism, continues to play a key role as a predictor variable in AIDS research. Our published work critiquing this thinking has typically taken on the form of a series of questions, some of which were presented in a 1998 commentary.

> First, if racism is a principal factor organizing social life, why not study racism rather than race? Second, why use an unscientific system of classification in scientific research? For racial classification systems are developed only when "race" is accepted as a legitimate variable. Why continue to accept something that is not only without biological merit but also full of evil social import? (Fullilove 1998)

The fact remains, however, that Americans are accustomed to viewing the world through the prism of race. The fact that HIV infection is sexually transmitted, or is spread through drug use, or is most likely to be prevalent in poor communities of color, seems consistent with our national beliefs about the way in which poverty and race function in America. Americans are accustomed to reading research reports and newspaper articles that confirm the view that, in addition to being mired in poverty, blacks and Latinos are less likely to score well on standardized tests of academic achievement, are less likely to go to college, are less likely to graduate if they do, are more likely to commit crimes, are more likely to go to prison, are more likely to contract a sexually transmitted disease, are more likely to have high blood pressure, asthma, diabetes, and be obese, and finally, are more likely to die before reaching the age of 65.

The data to support each of these assertions are massive. The association between race and health or race and social status is extremely powerful. What is subject to debate and dispute, however, are the answers to the questions, "Why does this happen, and what does it all mean?"

Race and AIDS: The View from the Inside

These "facts" about race take on their own significance within the affected communities, and, not surprisingly, so do the explanations as to why people of color are so terribly disadvantaged. The advent of the HIV/AIDS epidemic has been seen by many as just another chapter in the tragic history of assaults on the health and well-being of people of color. Frequently, when the topic is raised, the response comes back, "It's part of the conspiracy to wipe us all out!"

Our colleague, Michael Poulson (who is completing his doctoral dissertation at Columbia University, examining the role of myths and contemporary legends in the AIDS epidemic among people of color), has spent a number of years talking to blacks and Latinos about "The AIDS Conspiracy." The details of the conspiracy vary, but they all have essentially the same moral: that AIDS is a part of a larger plot to rid the nation of minorities and gay people. The origin of the virus is a central feature of conspiracy tales. Some theories hold that the epidemic is the result of failed biological warfare experiments. Others hold that HIV is actually a mutant version of a smallpox vaccine that was being tried out in Africa and got away from its creators. Other versions locate the conspiracy within the Pentagon, the CIA, the Trilateral Commission, the Office of the President of the United States, and/or various unnamed, shadowy government agencies. Many simply create various permutations and combinations of "all of the above." Still others hold that HIV is not even the cause of AIDS. What is killing people, they assert, are the drugs that people are being given to treat this so-called illness.

The strength of these beliefs is reflected in both casual conversation as well as in national polls. Survey research over the years has consistently demonstrated that significant numbers of African Americans believe that HIV/AIDS is indeed part of a racist plot to rid the nation of "undesireables." The public discourse on this topic is pervasive. Ask residents of the black or Latino communities in New York City to answer the question, "What do you hear about the 'true' origins of AIDS?" and, we would predict, in more than 90 percent of the responses, there will be some mention of one or more variations on a conspiracy motif.

These beliefs are not simply colorful, exotic bits of folklore in minority communities. We believe—as so many of our colleagues have asserted, from Stephen Thomas (Thomas & Quinn 1991) to Harlon Dalton (Dalton 1989)—that these views influence every effort that is mounted to alert community members to the threat of HIV and to act upon this threat. The impact is especially strong on programs that seek to have members of these communities get tested to learn about their HIV status or, if infected, to accept treatment with some of the new, powerful anti-HIV medications. Significantly, a recent recommendation to report the names of all persons with a positive HIV test to the CDC was viewed with particular suspicion. The official explanation— that such reporting would permit a more accurate means of tracking the course of the epidemic—was greeted with a snort by one participant in a HIV/AIDS Taskforce meeting in the Bronx. "Once they got your name in a computer, they own your life. You been bagged and tagged."

"Bagged and tagged"—meaning one is both infected with the virus and identified somewhere in a government computer database—neatly sums up the depths of suspicion about officially sponsored programs and initiatives to mobilize the community against HIV. A community resident need not have a deep, fundamental conviction that some version of a particular conspiracy tale is true. One need only be suspicious.

If the result of such belief or suspicion is inaction, the outcomes can vary from a failure to follow a recommended course of action (e.g., get tested or take a prescribed course of therapy) to an avoidance of physicians and clinical settings. Significantly, even community members who are infected with the virus and who are working to prevent its spread run the risk of being perceived as "sell outs" or as dupes of the very conspiracy that ensnared them in the first place.

Patricia Turner (1993), in her careful study of the role of myth and legend in African American life, has demonstrated that the two horns of this dilemma—belief in conspiracies on the one hand and widespread suspicion and mistrust of the white establishment on the other—have roots in the earliest contacts between Europeans and Africans. She writes:

> When the fully clothed Englishmen and the sparsely dressed Africans looked at each other, they came to the first of a long series of mutual misunderstandings— misunderstandings that may have permanently discolored their relationship. Each group needed to reconcile the foreign appearance and unfathomable actions of the other. And in trying to fit these unfamiliar "others" into their own worldview, both groups came to the same conclusion: these other people were cannibals.

Turner points out that the belief that the "other" group practiced cannibalism arose from mutual unfamiliarity. Black Africans were so unlike their European counterparts that Europeans frequently described blacks as "wild" or as "animals." The belief that wild, untamed, semi-human beasts would also eat other human beings was consistent with the notion that creatures lacking the taming influence of civilization would know no boundaries, including the most elemental boundaries about what can and cannot be eaten. Such beliefs about Africans made it easier, Turner notes, for Europeans to justify slavery. In such a worldview the selling of one human being to another is similar to selling a beast of burden. The denial of any claim to humanity on the part of the person being sold removes many, if not all, of the moral and ethical obligations that a civilized society would impose on the actions of the seller.

Africans, by contrast, struggled to make sense of the loss of large numbers of their family members and neighbors who were known to be herded into boats, taken out to sea, and never seen again. She writes:

> Having been forced to leave a familiar environment and to board enormous seafaring vessels, the Africans might certainly conclude that the fate awaiting them was not the kind of servitude they would have experienced as war booty in Africa. Massive-scale labor economies like the ones they were destined for in the New World were uncommon in Africa .... What else could the white man want but to eat them?

Turner points out that the legacy of this era remains in African American communities today. At issue, she maintains, is the degree to which the fate of the entire black community is tied to the fate of each and every black body. Mistrust about the "true" intentions of whites represents an important survival mechanism. Every act, every gesture, every pronouncement from mainstream society is judged, she asserts, by the degree to which it may be masking sinister intentions. There is an ineluctable logic to the attitudes community members will adopt to ensure their survival. It will take the form of a series of propositions such as this: to survive in a social system (a "democracy") that once enslaved you, that periodically submitted your community to the tender mercies of mob violence for hundreds of years without any reprisals to mob members, and that now throws as many as a third of your young men into prison each year, one must doubt everything.

Turner's most important contribution to our understanding of myths, rumors and conspiracy theories is the observation that for African Americans to be suspicious of the motives of larger American society is, after all, consistent with the evidence. Slavery, lynchings, mob rule, the Ku Klux Klan, excess infant mortality rates, high rates of HIV infection, and so on are, indeed, facts of life. Where, in the face of these facts, is the evidence that mainstream America has the best interests of African Americans (or other minority groups) at heart? Turner writes:

> Today, the political climate, for the most part, condemns overt attacks on black bodies. Evidence of covert violence, however, is easy to find. Black elected officials are drummed out of office; previously unknown diseases and devastatingly potent drugs decimate whole communities of blacks.
>
> As some African Americans attempt to reconcile the contradictions implicit in these signs, they embrace the familiar notion that the dominant culture remains intent on destroying blacks—one body at a time.

TRUTH VS. TRUST

Health educators and public health professionals often confront questions about the AIDS conspiracy in public meetings with members of minority communities. In the course of describing the benefits of an AIDS drug trial, or an initiative to increase the number of community residents who are tested for HIV antibodies, or in discussing the benefits of a new set of anti-HIV drugs, comments from audience members will sometimes question the conventional wisdom about the true nature of AIDS.

The knee-jerk reaction has been to dismiss these "non-facts" by supplying, in their stead, a set of "true facts." The unspoken assumption in this and in numerous other attempts to educate the public is that bits of information are interchangeable and that the falsities can easily be replaced by truths.

The reality is that—following Turner's reasoning—we are actually confronting deeply held belief systems for which simple acts of "fact replacement" will not suffice. The following "thought experiment" might help to make this clear:

> Imagine a devout, born-again Christian whose faith is so profound, he tithes.

Imagine that this individual is given a pamphlet in the course of a stroll in his community and that this pamphlet describes the life of the Prophet Mohammed. Suppose it contains approximately 800 words, contains a few colorful pictures, and has a layout not unlike that of a standard public health pamphlet designed to educate readers about AIDS.

Imagine that our Christian reader, immediately upon completing the reading of this pamphlet, converts, on the spot, to the faith of Islam. Now ask yourself: what are the odds of this happening?

The intent of the experiment is to convey how unlikely it is for people to change their beliefs, particularly deeply held beliefs, after a brief confrontation with a set of ostensibly contradictory "facts." The facts about HIV/AIDS are not self-evident. When individuals are confronted with contradictory information, it is often the credibility and authority invested in the fact-giver (not the facts themselves) that will determine what will be accepted as true and what will be rejected as false. It is a question of trust.

The authority vested in science is unquestioned by most Americans. It is the source of faith and truth in the modern age. It is at times almost impossible for us to imagine that science's hegemony in determining matters of truth would ever be questioned. However, this faith is why health educators and public health professionals have failed to recognize the significance and the tenacity of persistent myths and rumors about AIDS in poor communities of color (or even, it should be remembered, in communities of well-educated, white gay men).

WHAT IS TO BE DONE?

The resolution of this dilemma involves more than determining who is authorized to declare the "truth about AIDS." Rather, it lies in acknowledgement that what we have here—in those memorable words from the movie "Cool Hand Luke"—is a failure to communicate. At the core of the failure to get past suspicions that HIV is, indeed, fundamentally about the destruction of minority communities is the perception that the victim is being blamed.

Much of the focus for mainstream HIV/AIDS-related research and HIV/AIDS prevention campaigns is on individual risk taking. Public health research focuses on discovering the antecedents of HIV risk behavior and translating research results into "culturally competent" messages about who is at risk and who is not, and, more importantly, about what behaviors must be either avoided or embraced to protect against infection. The ultimate message here is often perceived as "AIDS is about you and what you do."

However, since the inception of the epidemic, the dominant strategy for giving this message salience has been to link it to data suggesting that non-whites are more likely to be infected than whites. It has typically been justified as the most efficient, obvious way of getting those at risk to sit up and pay attention.

Instead of digesting these facts and concluding, "Oh, I'm at risk. I need to take care," the response to this news has also included the question, "Why is this happening to me and my community more than it's affecting you guys?" As we have noted previously, HIV is simply being added to the list of problems that are unique to minority communities. The fact that suspicions about the origins of the AIDS crisis are routinely ignored or dismissed has meant that, for many, the threat of the epidemic has been obscured by the larger question: Is this all part of a larger plot to get us? Is it any wonder, therefore, that many of our attempts to mobilize affected communities have been ineffective?

We would maintain, moreover, that the failure of AIDS epidemiologic research to go beyond its heavy focus on race only adds fuel to this fire. We began this chapter by suggesting that such research is ultimately futile if it does not provide us with clues as to how affected individuals and communities can effectively combat the threat posed by the epidemic. Worse still, the impact of such research is that it appears to blame the victim—AIDS is your fault because you are engaged in all of this risky behavior—and fails to look at the social processes that victimize, or weaken wills, or that require heroic resistance and elastic resiliency.

Perhaps the greatest difficulty getting our colleagues and our students to accept the notion that racism, rather than race, is the key to understanding why AIDS has affected minority communities is that it requires a shift in the national dialogue about who and what is responsible for AIDS. It involves conceding that some of the premises for the conspiracy theories that AIDS researchers and public health professionals have so routinely dismissed as absurd have some basis in fact. It involves accepting the notion that being black or brown in America is hazardous for your health, and that our national failure to address the structural problems of race and poverty is partly responsible for the devastation of the AIDS epidemic.

Ours is by no means a new point of view. In an article published in 1989, entitled "AIDS In Blackface," Harlon Dalton, an African American professor of law at Yale and then a member of the National Commission on AIDS, sought to explain why the AIDS epidemic was not being "owned" by the black community, despite the obvious devastation it was beginning to wreak on people of color during the 1980s. He cites the fear of being blamed for the epidemic as one reason: "So long as we African Americans continue to worry that any hint of connection with AIDS will be turned against us, we will remain leery of accepting responsibility for its impact on our community."

More importantly, however, Dalton calls attention to the suspicion—prevalent a decade ago—that AIDS represents a genocidal threat. The longer the national failure to acknowledge that minority communities have a right to be concerned about this threat to community survival, the more these concerns are deemed to be valid. He is clear, as are we, that viewed through the eyes of community residents, there are reasons for these concerns. He writes:

> Two assumptions underlie the strong claim of genocide. The first is that the hostility of white America toward black America is so powerful, or the disregard so profound, that no depredation is unthinkable. This view is rooted in racial strife and feeds on the storehouse of sins visited upon blacks by whites. The second assumption is that under the right circumstances, the government is not above compromising the lives of innocent citizens. The grist for such a view is considerable.

The 90s have done little to blunt the impact of Dalton's observations. As he predicted, the 90s have, indeed, seen a shift in the epidemic from predominantly white to predominantly black and brown. Each newspaper headline proclaiming the increasing toll that AIDS is taking on communities of color only adds to the belief that the threat to community life is real. The failure to acknowledge the legitimacy of community concerns that "this is more than just a public health issue" undoubtedly only heightens the suspicion with which each new AIDS program is received.

The community's agenda about what needs doing is quite long and deals with issues that are often seen as more immediate and pressing than HIV/AIDS. It includes dealing with the lack of jobs and housing. It includes concerns about crime (as well as the high rates of imprisonment of the community's young men) and concerns about the police. In New York City, these concerns are more strongly connected to HIV than one might initially suspect. The high crime and arrest rates stem largely from the fallout from the sale and use of illicit drugs. The relationship between drug use and HIV needs no elaboration, but the role of drug dealing in filling the vacuum created when job opportunities fled the inner city is critical. From there the link between jobs, crime, drug use and drug sales, and HIV/AIDS is not difficult to establish.

The increase in the prison population also has direct impact on this relationship. The high rates of HIV infection in the prisons and the circulation of HIV-infected men and women between high HIV seroprevalence communities and high HIV seroprevalence jails is arguably one of the most effective engines for maintaining a reservoir of infection imaginable. This same engine also provides the means to expose an ever-growing number of community residents to risk, either in the jails themselves or in the communities whose residents fill the jails.

This view of the epidemic is not a significant part of the current national dialogue on AIDS among researchers, policy makers, health educators, public health professionals, or the students who are training to enter these professions. As we have tried to suggest in this essay, these are not simply exotic, ancillary issues in understanding the impact of HIV/AIDS on poor communities of color. Placing them in the forefront of the issues that we deal with in designing interventions for these communities is vital. Encouraging a national dialogue that acknowledges these realities may just be the most important first step we can take to halt the sobering realities of the growing HIV/AIDS epidemic.

References for this essay may be found on page 150.

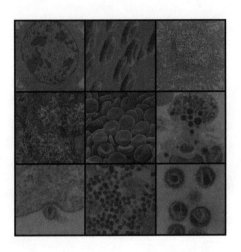

EIGHT

HIV/AIDS AND INSTITUTIONAL TRANSFORMATION:
THE EXPERIENCE OF SAN FRANCISCO STATE UNIVERSITY

Robert A. Corrigan and Sheila A. McClear
SAN FRANCISCO STATE UNIVERSITY

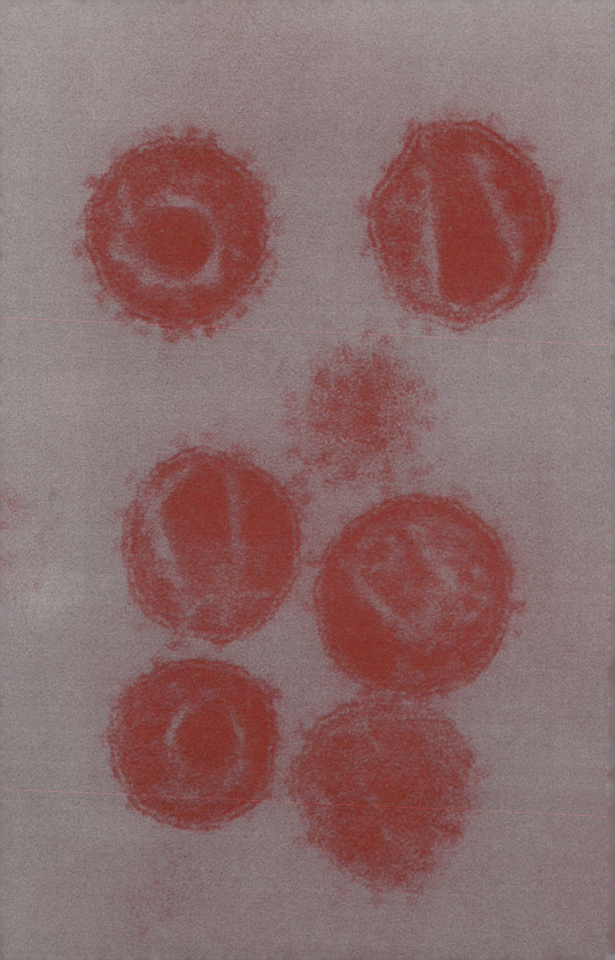

San Francisco State University's engagement with the HIV/AIDS crisis began much as it probably did on many other campuses: with the discovery in 1982 that a member of the campus community—a staff member, in SF State's case—had AIDS. So little was then known about the disease that some of the employee's colleagues were actually concerned about using the same telephones. Education about the realities of prevention and transmission thus became the university's first, urgent need. Policies and practices would need to come next, as would a more complex and integrated approach to a life issue that soon touched every part of the campus community.

What no one could possibly have predicted in 1982 was the way San Francisco State's HIV/AIDS response would, over the next seventeen years, expand, evolve, and mature into a tightly-woven academic/student affairs/human resources/community relations effort that has made the university stronger as an educational institution and as an academic community.

It is no exaggeration to call the overall effect of the campus response to HIV/AIDS transformational. Thanks to a number of passionately dedicated people, to widespread administrative support, and to an approach that from the start encouraged linkages between parts of the university that traditionally operate fairly separately (e.g. academic affairs and student affairs; students and administrators), SFSU's HIV/AIDS response has become—as crises can—a unifying force. It is a point of campus-wide pride, a reinforcer of key university values, and an interdisciplinary vehicle for learning. It has changed lives and opened minds.

SFSU's response is also a work in progress. As knowledge of and treatment for AIDS has advanced, as the demographics of the disease have changed, and as AIDS has become old news to some, the campus program has had to adapt, developing ways to fight compassion fatigue, complacency, and the sense of diminished risk bred of powerful new medications.

Some will wonder whether the experiences of this University, set in a particularly progressive city that was ground zero for the epidemic, are likely to be broadly translatable. We strongly believe that they are. We have drawn on the same resources of knowledge and caring that are present on all campuses. Furthermore, for institutions located in communities that have developed fewer health and other support systems for people with HIV/AIDS than has San Francisco, the need is even greater to offer students, staff, faculty, and the greater community itself the full range of education and support that may be hard to obtain off the campus.

San Francisco State University's response to HIV/AIDS since 1982 can be divided into three periods, each marked by its particular concerns and achievements; each serving to transform the campus community.

THE EARLY YEARS: EDUCATION AND PREVENTION

Milestones:

- SFSU presents the AIDS Prevention Project, a week-long conference

- The AIDS Coordinating Committee is formally established

- The university's AIDS policy is enacted

- Education programs are created and expanded

- The study of AIDS begins to appear in the curriculum

- An AIDS education supplement, "Playing It Safe," appears regularly in the student newspaper and elsewhere on campus

Between 1982 and, roughly, 1988, the need for education about a still poorly understood disease was the driving force behind SFSU's AIDS effort. A February 1988 feature on "AIDS and the University" in the university newsletter noted that "Attitudes toward AIDS have changed on campus during the past two years." Credit for the change was given to a ground-breaking conference, the first of its kind in the California State University system, perhaps the first nationally or even internationally. This was a week-long AIDS Prevention Project, held in fall of 1985, open to the entire community, and drawing attendees from as far away as Finland. With a frankness that would only later become common, panels discussed transmission, testing for the virus, and safe sex.

The *ad hoc* task force that had formed to present the conference achieved official status several months later as the AIDS Coordinating Committee (ACC), charged with the responsibility for mounting educational programs. A separate steering committee was established to recommend campus policy. The ACC included faculty, students, and staff and, in its first year, sponsored more than 140 education events, including classes, information sessions for employees, a speakers bureau, videos, workshops, and a host of publications.

The University enacted its first official AIDS policy in 1986, guaranteeing the rights of students and employees with AIDS to work, study, and use all campus facilities. The policy was to become a model for the California State University System. Curricular connections were made with a clinical science professor offering a course on AIDS (believed to be the first such class offered for credit on a U.S. campus), a health educator developing or revising two classes, and a biology professor creating a new course: The Biology of a Modern Epidemic (still taught). Work began on a general education (core curriculum) option on AIDS for the culminating "relationships of knowledge" segment.

With campus policy in place and education programs reaching from classroom to dorm room, the university was ready to take the next step: institutionalizing its AIDS response.

THE MIDDLE YEARS: MAINTAINING ENERGY, ENSURING CONTINUATION

Milestones:

- The AIDS Coordinating Committee becomes a regular budget item

- The campus Memorial Grove is opened

- Campus donations—many through payroll deduction—establish the Kolb Fund to provide grants usable for any purpose to SFSU students, faculty, or staff with HIV/AIDS

- Students, faculty, and staff design and sew an SFSU section for the national AIDS quilt

- The student health center begins to offer anonymous, low-cost HIV testing

- University AIDS policy is revised to include HIV and reference to the Americans With Disabilities Act (ADA)

- HIV/AIDS curriculum expands in number of courses and disciplines

- Employee policies evolve—catastrophic leave is added

In the fall of 1988, Robert A. Corrigan arrived at San Francisco State University as president to find a campus already deeply engaged with an issue that had scarcely begun to register on the east coast campus he had just left. He often cites the statistic quoted to him by then-San Francisco Mayor Art Agnos: "More San Franciscans have died of AIDS than in all U.S. wars since California joined the Union." SFSU's AIDS response, largely a dedicated volunteer effort up to now, needed institutional stability and support. In the next few years, the AIDS Coordinating Committee was made a regular university budget item and release time was provided for its chair, in recognition of a growing workload. The AIDS policy was updated, adding reference to HIV and the Americans with Disabilities Act.

SFSU also provided support and funding for what has proved to be a very important ACC project: the creation of the Memorial Grove in a beautiful campus site, as a place where those the university community had lost could be celebrated and remembered. Though AIDS prompted the creation of the grove, the site is deliberately inclusive in name and use. Recently, for example, a service was held there for a young athlete who died of a heart problem. The Grove evokes a sense of community and provides a place for the university community to share its losses—all losses. Such inclusiveness emerged from the HIV/AIDS response, and has been critical to its sustained success.

The creation of an SFSU section for the national Names Project quilt brought a dedicated group together for hundreds of hours of work on a beautiful set of panels that included the names of all those the university community had so far lost to AIDS. Those who worked on the quilt ended by feeling closer to each other—believing, too, that they were a part of the campus HIV/AIDS effort.

Increasingly, the campus community wanted to help its own, and an unusual new fund gave them a way. The Cindy Kolb Fund, named for the popular director of Disabled Student Services, who had just died (not of AIDS), provides grants to faculty, students, and staff with HIV/AIDS. It is singular in two respects: The awards can be used for any purpose, from textbooks to emergency expenses to new clothes, and faculty and staff can contribute through payroll deduction. The university waives accounting charges. So far, more than $120,000 has been distributed.

Because of concerns about confidentiality, the ACC postponed campus HIV/AIDS testing. When the ACC and Student Health Services (SHS) were confident that anonymity could be maintained, SHS began, in 1994, to offer low-cost ($9) tests.

People were, by now, living longer with AIDS, and SFSU took another look at its benefit policies, to see what could reasonably be done to help those who were exhausting their sick leave. The catastrophic leave plan which was developed allows university employees to donate portions of their earned sick leave to a central pool, administered by the human resources department for the benefit of ill colleagues. Faculty, staff, and administrators have responded generously over the years.

Curricular engagement expanded greatly. Faculty still requested guest lecturers through ACC, but in a significant development, more faculty were now integrating HIV/AIDS into their classes themselves. By 1994, about sixty courses included an HIV/AIDS component.

The net effect of these projects of the middle years cannot be measured by dollars raised or leave hours donated. The real and lasting value has been the much broader sense of common effort and community that emerged. As the number of people who were engaged in some way with the university's HIV/AIDS effort steadily increased, the community became more compassionate, more thoughtful, and more united. To be sure, an important unifying characteristic is that there is probably not a single member of the campus community who has not lost a partner, relative, friend, or colleague to AIDS.

When a much-loved staff member was critically ill with AIDS, for example, a support group of some twenty-five campus colleagues quickly formed. They took turns bringing dinner to his home and spending the night with him; one had his power-of-attorney; another provided nutritional counseling. All were with him to the end. As Hollis Matson, a health educator and one of the founders of the ACC, said, "It was a terrific community effort, and it resulted in a lot of us staying in AIDS work in one way or another."

This new feeling of connectedness did not stop at the edge of campus. A university team of faculty, students, and staff took on a regular Project Open Hand route, delivering hot meals to people in the city with HIV/AIDS. The effort continues to this day.

In the fall of 1994, *The Chronicle of Higher Education* published a cover story on San Francisco State's AIDS response. Biology faculty member Ann Auleb, who had been a leader from the very start in developing academic and informational programs, told the reporter that "the real story" was the way the campus had come together because of AIDS. Increasingly, we were recognizing the transformation in ourselves.

THE MID-90S AND BEYOND: BROADENING PARTNERSHIPS, INCREASING STUDENT INVOLVEMENT, ADAPTING TO CHANGE

Milestones:

- The AIDS Coordinating Committee chair becomes a funded, permanent university position

- Curricular ties broaden

- Peer education programs engage many more students; students turn to the Web

- Student focus groups help AIDS Coordinating Committee learn and test new strategies

- Campus health and sexuality services work as a partnership

- A holistic approach links HIV/AIDS education with substance abuse

- Education strategies adapt to new AIDS demographics, new social attitudes

Last year, San Francisco State University successfully completed a two-year, grass-roots strategic planning effort, which began with six planning themes: academic excellence, teaching and learning success, the user-friendly campus, internationalizing the curriculum, community responsibility, and combating discrimination. Though the university's HIV/AIDS response began long before this strategic plan was conceived, it is easy to see that it addresses every one of those themes.

That is pretty good assurance that the university has developed something that will endure. It is also reassurance: HIV/AIDS activities at SFSU should endure; they are appropriate—even central—to the campus community, and they advance its mission. As Richard Keeling puts it: "Education about HIV/AIDS is education for life."

The subject of HIV/AIDS itself has broad curricular ramifications—health and medicine, of course, but also public policy, economics, psychology, ethics, international relations, the arts, literature, ethnic studies, and more. Discussion of HIV/AIDS from any perspective fosters key intellectual skills: critical thinking; viewing a complex problem from many perspectives; gathering and weighing evidence; analyzing cause and effect, and communicating effectively to multiple audiences. This subject provides an unparalleled starting point for academic work.

San Francisco State faculty clearly agree. HIV/AIDS is integrated into the curriculum in many of the expected academic areas: clinical science, biology, nursing, counseling, health education, psychology. But faculty are also weaving it into mathematics, philosophy, statistics, history, Black studies, art history, and international relations. A Russian language course on the Russian press includes a segment on sexuality, including AIDS. A math instructor uses false positive/false negative HIV antibody tests results to illustrate conditional probability. And a history professor draws analogies to the AIDS epidemic in classes which touch on the Black Death and the impact of disease on Native American populations.

In and outside the classroom, engagement with HIV/AIDS has helped SFSU toward its goal of providing a campus climate in which all can flourish—embracing diversity and combating all forms of discrimination. Many faculty say that the classroom discussion of HIV/AIDS changed their students, and them. With students who often knew more about AIDS than their professors, the professor became less the magisterial expert and more the co-learner.

In the classroom, people began to talk—and listen—who otherwise might never have engaged with each other at all, much less so frankly. AIDS caused a conversation. The conversation didn't necessarily make students into friends, but, says Hollis Matson, "more important, it got people to hear each other's words and see each other's feelings."

SFSU's AIDS response also enhanced its diversity efforts. In the early years, AIDS was viewed as a disease of white homosexual males. But as time went on, more and more people from other racial and ethnic groups, as well as women, came to see AIDS as their issue, too. At ACC meetings, a conference table mostly of white faces changed to a gathering much more reflective of the university's diversity. People who had previously stayed in their separate groups found themselves working together. In this way, too, the conversation broadened.

The university's new strategic plan commits us to becoming a more "user-friendly" university. Breaking down artificial barriers between administrative areas in order to unify services and simplify procedures is one of our key strategies. Here too, the AIDS effort has moved forward, creating powerful new partnerships. Student affairs, student government, academic affairs, and the student health center work together on HIV/AIDS-related educational and service programs. The human resources department, part of the team since the beginning, counsels faculty as well as staff and administrators on all the classroom and workplace issues HIV/AIDS raises. With faculty support, student health services offers a series of credit-bearing workshops on health education topics, including several on HIV and AIDS. The chair of the AIDS Coordinating Committee, student affairs counseling professional Michael Ritter, teaches a 6-unit class to train peer counselors for participation in HIV/AIDS education and referral programs both on and off campus, emphasizing "active learning," service learning, and community service. The university's HIV/AIDS response has strengthened all three. A few examples demonstrate the range and value of student-led (and often classroom-linked) activities.

For the last five years, students have staffed a peer education booth at the student center. Others give presentations to residence hall students—probably the youngest cohort on campus, hence a higher-risk group—to classes (at faculty request), and to student organizations. Statistics show a rise in AIDS among women and in communities of color, and so, with Ritter's assistance, peer educators have over the last year conducted student focus groups based on cultural, sexual, disability, and gender diversity. What they are learning will help design and target effective prevention efforts for various communities. Students now organize and present the campus' Multicultural AIDS Day, while the ACC provides the funding. Responding to student requests for an entirely private, yet frank source of information about HIV/AIDS and campus services, several SFSU students created "Web Peers," an internet site that allows students to submit questions anonymously, (answered on-line by ACC members and university health educators). Anyone can access the site (www.sfsu.edu/~aidsinfo/Peer/).

One of the best of SFSU's new approaches to HIV/AIDS education is the deliberate inclusion of HIV education into programs aimed at preventing alcohol abuse and drug use. These programs recognize, for example, that alcohol abuse can lead not only to acquaintance rape, but to unsafe sex, whether consensual or not, and thus to sexually transmitted diseases, including HIV. In this way, students get a message that HIV/AIDS is not a "them" issue, but an "everybody" concern.

Instead of fading, as they are reported to have done on many campuses, peer education activities are burgeoning at San Francisco State. They may, in fact, be its best new strategy in an always-changing effort to increase AIDS awareness. "The biggest crisis we're facing now is a feeling that HIV/AIDS is over," says Ritter. Studies show that AIDS is on the rise again among young people in their teens and early 20s, yet many students believe that because of powerful new medications, they no longer have to fear the infection. Ritter and his colleagues have found, as have several studies of successful drug education programs, that peers have powerful voices. And students who discover their power are primed to be a force for good, active in their communities throughout their lives.

Over these years, SFSU has seen some welcome changes. The Kolb Fund now receives requests for books and fees, things that imply a future, rather than, as in early days, money to take a caretaker out to dinner, or to go home to say goodbye to family. The new Bob Westwood Scholarship Fund was created for the student with HIV or AIDS who is thinking about the long term, about a career path.

Other changes are more difficult. Such a supportive environment has been established that the university now occasionally must deal with employees who are really too ill to work, yet want to stay on the job, and with those employees' troubled, sympathetic supervisors. In these cases, Human Relations Director Denise Fox works one-on-one with the supervisor and employee on the appropriate steps and support. This is a small price to pay for a great overall good. As Fox notes, "Prior to AIDS, we had rigid protocols about how and when people worked, and we were not open to change. Now we are much more creative in responding to individual needs and balancing them against organizational requirements." The change has helped not just those with HIV/AIDS, but all people on campus with disabilities.

There is more to SFSU's HIV/AIDS response than has been laid out here, and many, many more people who made it happen than have been mentioned. Still, this is a reasonably full portrait of what HIV/AIDS has done to—and for—this campus. Because of their HIV/AIDS response, administrators, faculty, and staff have cut across boundaries to come together in a common effort. They have enriched the curriculum, tied education to life in powerful ways, given students a range of new opportunities for responsibility and active learning, strengthened their ties to the community beyond the campus, and, perhaps most important of all, come to feel a shared pride in this multi-faceted and still-evolving effort.

Out of an initial effort to cope with a terrible disease has come something more deeply tied to the university's educational and social mission.

The current status of the organization that started it all, the AIDS Coordinating Committee, is further indication that the University has been permanently and positively altered. Today, fourteen years after its founding, the ACC is a recognized, respected, and administratively supported center of HIV/AIDs efforts. Once *ad hoc*, with no administrative charge or home, it is now fully institutionalized, reporting to—and receiving budgetary support from—the vice president for student affairs, with a salaried chair, campuswide visibility, and excellent ties with the faculty, student support units, and with students themselves, both individually and through student organizations. The steering committee, a group drawn from the ACC and others, and appointed by the president, continues to propose, assess, and help implement SFSU's HIV/AIDS policy.

San Francisco State has been successful in forging a response to HIV/AIDS because, from the start, the AIDS effort was inclusive, holistic, and good at involving a growing number of members of the campus community in ways that fit their university roles and responsibilities. Higher education institutions cannot exist in a vacuum—every campus needs community ties and partnerships. They have the capacity and, it is arguable, the obligation to be value leaders, as well as knowledge leaders. All this comes together powerfully in HIV/AIDS. There is no doubt that San Francisco State University is a sadder community because of HIV/AIDS, but it is also a better one.

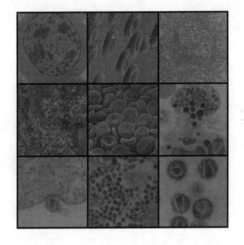

RESOURCES

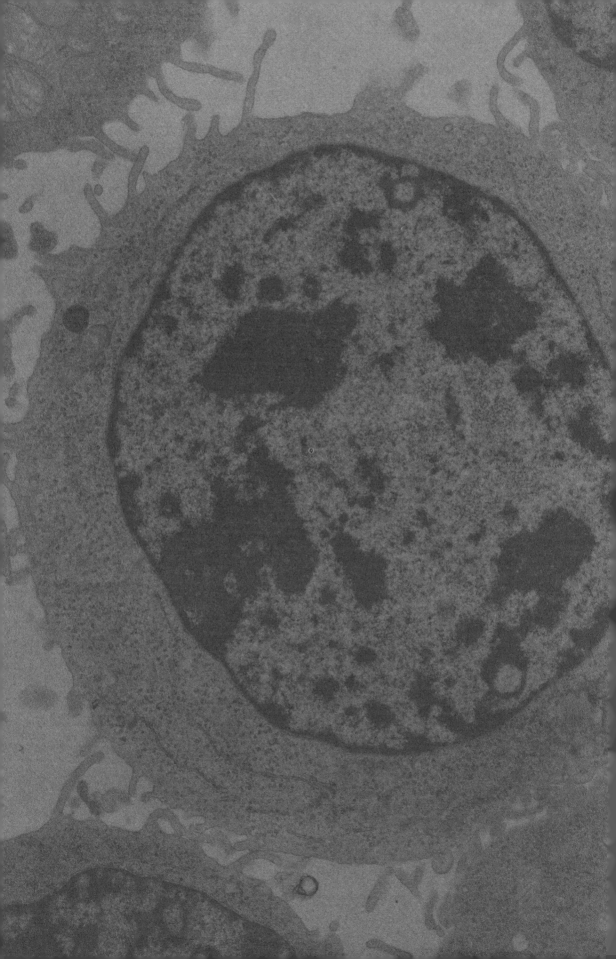

How to Use This Book....

While we think that *Learning for Our Common Health* is an attractive book, we hope that this copy will neither just decorate an office nor live out its life as a forgotten resident on a bookshelf somewhere.

We envision and intend multiple uses for this "foundational" monograph. Here are a few suggestions for using this book with particular campus constituencies and for particular campus purposes:

For leadership retreats and strategic planning: The monograph contains useful materials to help colleges and universities include health and attention to HIV/AIDS in their comprehensive efforts to address matters of importance to students and the communities in which colleges and universities are located. Corrigan and McClear specifically relate this work to campus strategic planning. Cronon's essay provides a useful framework for a discussion of general and liberal education. For campuses interested in better integrating academic and student affairs initiatives, Keeling's analysis will be helpful. All of the essays provide provocative and useful bases for discussions and, in many instances, they contain or imply "standards" against which a campus' efforts may be compared and improvements charted.

For faculty and student use in undergraduate classes: All of these materials contain important arguments and insights that will prove useful to pre-professional education in a variety of fields. For example: The Cronon essay on what it means to be educated would be especially useful as a text for organizing discussions in freshman and first-year programs and in capstone experiences. The Bell and Fullilove essays provide valuable material for students in ethics, public policy, diversity initiatives, and a host of academic programs. And those studying leadership will be particularly interested in Reed's essay.

For campus HIV/AIDS task forces and committees to assist in their work, including their advocacy for improved efforts: All of the essays should be useful to those who are charged with focusing a campus' attention and some of its resources on HIV/AIDS and student and community health. Especially noteworthy and useful for these groups should be the essay by Keeling, which suggests a re-framing of our understanding of health, the piece by Bell, which offers a moral justification for interest in and actions on these issues, and that of Harkavy and Romer, who suggest ways of improving engagement with the community. The Corrigan and McClear essay traces a development path that campuses may choose to follow and reaches an outcome that others may wish to emulate.

For curriculum planners and groups charged with improving educational outcomes: Supplementing the analyses and philosophical justifications provided by Cronon, Keeling, and Bell, Harkavy and Romer offer concrete suggestions for service learning in support of academic objectives. The Partner Institutions listed in the resource section and the PHHE program itself can and will provide useful individual models of curricular engagement with HIV/AIDS.

For members of campus governing boards: Reed's essay on leadership and the Cronon essay outline a set of benefits that can come from engagement with the many issues raised by HIV/AIDS and provide a useful background overview for board consideration. The pieces by Corrigan and McClear, Harkavy and Romer, the Fulliloves, and Keeling identify important links between higher education and the communities that support and depend on them.

For those engaged in campus diversity and anti-bigotry initiatives: All the authors pay attention to the connections between HIV and issues of human dignity and social justice. The essay by the Fulliloves should be especially helpful in informing and refreshing dialogues about race and health. Bell's piece on ethics locates important issues of education and its antithesis in the context of democratic and civic education.

For those seeking to develop deeper and more productive relationships with the community: The essay by Harkavy and Romer will be useful to those who are trying to locate a philosophical and pedagogical basis for service learning and has useful material for those evaluating and initiating programs. The Fulliloves provide important cautionary advice and suggest a heuristic strategy that could improve the chances for successful engagements with those who don't credit higher education with great face validity.

For graduate and professional students in the health disciplines, education, and higher education administration: All the essays should have some utility in graduate education. The pieces by Bell and the Fulliloves will be of use to those in teacher education and, with the piece by Keeling, should also help those studying in the health fields. The Keeling paper will also have utility in graduate classes preparing students for work in the area of student personnel services.

As this monograph goes to press, the Program for Health and Higher Education is deeply engaged in the development of a companion resource, The National Leadership Resource Database for Health and Higher Education. This will be a web-based, searchable interactive database designed to be an intensely practical complement to this foundational monograph. It will offer links to professors and particular courses, campus policies and programs, and other resources to support the development of this work. One feature we hope to design will be a series of expanded "guides" for how to use this monograph and to also post reports on how it is being used. Access to the database will be announced though the AAC&U website, at www.aacu-edu.org/initiatives.

Web-based Resources on HIV/AIDS and Health

The following are World Wide Web-based resources for information and statistics on HIV/AIDS and health. Since information and statistics about the pandemic change frequently, it is best to use these resources to locate the most current information.

- For information on HIV/AIDS and health in the United States, see the Centers for Disease Control and Prevention (CDC) website for Data and Statistics at:

  http://www.cdc.gov/scientific.htm

- For global information and statistics on HIV/AIDS and other sexually transmitted infections, see the World Health Organization (WHO) website at:

  http: //www who.int/asd

- For more information about the Program for Health and Higher Education (PHHE), see the Association of American Colleges and Universities (AAC&U) website at:

  http://www.aacu-edu.org/initiative/health.html

- The National Center for Chronic Disease Prevention and Health Promotion maintains a website for their Division of Adolescent and School Health (DASH) at:

  http://www.cdc.gov/nccdphp/dash

- For the entire report of the Youth Risk Behavior Surveillance: National College Health Risk Behavior Survey–United States, 1995, see:

  http://www.cdc.gov/nccdphp/dash/mmwrfile/ss4606.htm

- The National Center for HIV, STD, and TB Prevention maintains a website for their Division of HIV/AIDS Prevention at:

  http://www.cdc.gov/nchstp/hiv_aids/dhap.htm

PARTNERS IN HEALTH AND HIGHER EDUCATION

Partners in Health and Higher Education were selected following a competitive process in two cohorts in 1997-1998 and 1998-1999. Each received modest financial support to collaborate with PHHE and other partners and to pursue activities outlined in their applications. In addition to the PHHE National Partners, seven Maryland institutions were also designated as partners through the generous support of the Maryland Higher Education Commission. The partnership program is a leadership initiative that encourages the development of approaches that enhance individual campus efforts and offer models for diffusion and broad adaptation. Listed below are the names of the partner institutions and the contact persons who can provide details on the work undertaken to improve education and health:

Anna Maria College
Paxton, Massachussetts
Contact: Dr. Cynthia Patterson at 508/849-3359 or cpatters@anna-maria.edu

Beloit College
Beloit, Wisconsin
Contact: Dr. Marion Field Fass at 608/363-2784

Buffalo State College
Buffalo, New York
Contact: Dr. Gail Dinter-Gottlieb at 7016/878-6434 or dintergg@buffalostate.edu

City College of CUNY
New York, New York
Contact: Dr. Thomas Morales at 212/650-5426 or tdmcc@cunyvm.cuny.edu

The College of New Jersey
Hillwood Lakes, New Jersey
Contact: Dr. Laurie Sherwen at 609/771-2541 or sherwen@tcnj.edu

Jacksonville University
Jacksonville, Florida
Contact: Dr. Karen Jackson at 904/744-3950 ext. 7321 or kjackso@mail.ju.edu

Madonna University
Livonia, Michigan
Contact: Dr. James Copi at 313/432-5510 or copi@smtp.munet.edu or
Dr. Ernest Nolan at 313/432-5313

Millikin University
Decatur, Illinois
Contact: Ms. Deborah Slayton at 217/424-6366 or dlslayton@mail.millikin.edu

Prince George's Community College
Largo, Maryland
Contact: Ms. Edith Linville at 301/341-3034 or linville@erols.com

Rutgers University
New Brunswick, New Jersey
Contact: Dr. Godfrey Roberts at 932/932-8433 or roberts@fas-admin.rutgers.edu

Saint Francis College
Loretto, Pennsylvania
Contact: Ms. Martha O'Brien at 814/472-3111 or mobrien@sfcpa.edu

Southeast Missouri State University
Cape Girardeau, Missouri
Contact: Dr. Christina Fraser at 573/651-2384 or cfrazier@biology.semo.edu

State University of New York at Stony Brook
Stony Brook, New York
Contact: Dr. Helen Lemay at 516/632-7500 or hlemay@ccmail.sunysb.edu

Tennessee Technological University
Cookeville, Tennessee
Contact: Dr. Matthew Zagumny at 931/752-6255 or mzagumny@tntech.edu

The University of Arizona
Tucson, Arizona
Contact: Dr. Janice Monk at 520/621-7338 or jmonk@u.arizona.edu or
Dr. Sally Stevens at 520/749-7156 or sallys@azstarnet.com

The University of Kentucky
Lexington, Kentucky
Contact: Dr. Holly Riffe at 606/257-2665 or hariff@pop.uky.edu

The University of Massachusetts/Boston
Boston, Massachussetts
Contact: Dr. Amy Rex Smith at 617/287-7534 or rex_smith@umbsky.cc.umb.edu

Washington State University
Pullman, Washington
Contact: Dr. Thomas A. Brigham at 509/335-4634 or brigham@mail.wsu.edu

Wesleyan College
Macon, Georgia
Contact: Dr. Priscilla Danheiser at 912/757-5229 or
priscilla_danheiser@post.wesleyan-college.edu

Wesleyan University
Middleton, Connecticut
Contact: Dr. David L. Beveridge at 860/685-2575 or dbeveridge@wesleyan.edu

MARYLAND PARTNERSHIP INITIATIVE

Cecil Community College
North East, Maryland
Contact: Jane Sharrow at 410/287-6060, ext. 554 or jsharrow@ed.cecil.cc.md.us

Coppin State College
Baltimore, Maryland
Contact: Clayton McNeill at 410/383-5800 or d6pcvpl@coa.oppin.umd.edu

Frostburg State University
Frostburg, Maryland
Contact: John Lowe at 301/687-4226 or d2pclowe@fra00.fsu.umd.edu

Towson State University
Towson, Maryland
Contact: Jane Halpern at 410/830-2466 or jhalpern@towson.edu

University of Maryland, Baltimore
Baltimore, Maryland
Contact: Thomasine D. Guberski at 410/706-5712 or guberski@nurse-1.ab.umd.edu

University of Maryland, Baltimore County
Catonsville, Maryland
Contact: Mitzi Mabe at 410/455-4384 or mabe@umbc.edu

ASSOCIATION OF AMERICAN COLLEGES AND UNIVERSITIES
PROGRAM FOR HEALTH AND HIGHER EDUCATION

HIGHER EDUCATION, HIV, AND HEALTH:

A NATIONAL LEADERSHIP STATEMENT

As leaders of higher education, we are committed to improving education and the human condition. By fostering a broader engagement with issues of HIV and public health, we can do both. We can enrich liberal education, discover and test new strategies for curriculum integration, strengthen connections between academic and student life goals, and reduce the spread of HIV disease.

AIDS is a pressing societal problem, and the academy has clear civic and educational obligations to contribute to its solution. As a disease, AIDS is the leading cause of death in the United States of those between the ages of 25 and 44, and it is a critical international public health issue. Our students, as future leaders, will be required to understand, manage, and solve complex issues of health and their social and political implications. To reduce personal risk, students must acquire a comprehensive understanding of AIDS and a growing respect for their own health and the health of others.

Worthy of serious study as a part of the liberal education of any citizen, health and HIV are also powerful vehicles for student learning and curricular reform. They raise an unusually broad array of questions in many disciplines. Their study will encourage teaching and learning across boundaries to connect the campus with the community, the curriculum with the co-curriculum, the arts and sciences with the professional disciplines, and the arts and science disciplines with one another. They lend themselves well to active and experiential forms of student inquiry and learning, and to service learning both on campus and in the community.

We endorse the efforts of the U.S. Centers for Disease Control and Prevention to encourage a national strategy that engages higher education with issues of public health. We strongly support and pledge our assistance to our colleagues who are providing leadership to make health a more central concern of undergraduate education, and we call on others to do the same.

Adopted by the Board of Directors of the Association of American Colleges and Universities and by the National Leadership Advisory Board for the Program for Health and Higher Education, Fall 1997.

NATIONAL LEADERSHIP ADVISORY BOARD
PROGRAM FOR HEALTH AND HIGHER EDUCATION

Nora Kizer Bell
President
Wesleyan College

William E. Bennett
Senior Health Science Advisor to the
Secretary (Retired)
U.S. Department of Health and Human
Services

Robert A. Corrigan
President
San Francisco State University

Barbara Doherty
Director
Institute of Religious Formation
Catholic Theological Union

Gwendolyn Dungy
Executive Director
National Association of Student Personnel
Administrators

Peter Facione
Dean
College of Arts and Sciences
Santa Clara University

Patricia Florestano
Secretary of Higher Education
Maryland Higher Education Commission

John N. Gardner
Executive Director
National Resource Center for the Freshman
Year Experience
University of South Carolina

Ira Harkavy
Director
Center for Community Partnerships
University of Pennsylvania

Thomas K. Hearn, Jr.
President
Wake Forest University

Richard Keeling
Director
University Health Services
and Professor of Medicine
University of Wisconsin–Madison

Richard L. McCormick
President
University of Washington

Elizabeth McKinsey
Dean
Carleton College

Karen Kashmanian Oates
Professor
George Mason University

NOTES ON CONTRIBUTORS

NORA KIZER BELL is the first woman to be named president of Wesleyan College in Macon, Georgia, the first college in the world chartered to grant degrees to women. A philosopher by training, whose special interest is bioethics, Bell is the author of *Who Decides? Conflicts in Rights in Health Care*. From 1993-97, she was dean of the College of Arts and Sciences at the University of North Texas. Previously, she was professor of philosophy and director of the Center for Bioethics at the University of South Carolina, where her interests in HIV/AIDS led her to develop one of the first college courses on HIV. For her service to South Carolina, she received the Order of the Palmetto, the highest civilian award presented by the governor. Bell's baccalaureate degree is from Randolph Macon Woman's College, and her doctorate was earned at the University of North Carolina. She has served on the editorial board of AIDS Education and is now on the Georgia Health Decisions Board, the National Academy of Academic Leadership Advisory Board, and the Sun Trust Bank's board. Bell is currently at work on her second book, *Tyranny of the Majority*.

WM. DAVID BURNS directs the Program for Health and Higher Education at the Association of American Colleges and Universities. Burns's degrees are in political science, with a concentration in political theory, from Rutgers University. For more than twenty years he was a member of the administration at Rutgers, where he served as director of university health services and assistant vice president for student life policy and services. He is the author of *College, Alcohol and Choices, Ways to Go: Directions for HIV/AIDS Prevention on Our Nation's Campuses*, and *The Web of Caring* (with Margaret Klawunn). Burns founded the New Jersey Collegiate Consortium for Health and Education and in 1994 was appointed to the adjunct faculty of the Robert Wood Johnson School of Medicine. Governor Christine Whitman named him to her Juvenile Justice and Delinquency Prevention Advisory Committee in 1995.

ROBERT CORRIGAN has spent twenty years as an urban university president, first at the University of Massachusetts-Boston and since 1988 at San Francisco State University. A national leader in university community service and service learning initiatives, he was appointed by President Clinton to head the presidential steering group for "America Reads," and he was named by Education Secretary Riley to the steering committee for "America Goes Back to School." Corrigan also chairs California Campus Compact, a statewide arm of a national consortium of colleges and universities committed to a strong public service mission. He serves as co-chair of the Leadership Board of the Bay Area School Reform Collaborative–Annenberg Challenge, he is a member of the board of directors of the World Affairs Council, and he has served on the boards of the Private Industry Council of San Francisco and the Chamber of Commerce. A graduate of Brown University, Corrigan earned his doctorate in American Civilization from the University of Pennsylvania. He helped to develop the University of Iowa's first Black Studies program and produced the first extensive bibliography of African American fiction.

WILLIAM CRONON is Frederick Jackson Turner professor of history, geography, and environmental studies at the University of Wisconsin–Madison. Cronon's research is concerned with the ways human communities modify the landscapes in which they live and how people are in turn affected by changing geological, climatological, epidemiological, and ecological conditions. His books have won several prestigious prizes, including the Bancroft prize for *Nature's Metropolis: Chicago and the Great West.* Cronon serves as the general editor of the Weyerhaeuser Environmental Books Series for the University of Washington Press. In 1996, he became the director of the Honors Program for the College of Letters and Science, and more recently he has become the founding academic director of the Chadbourne Residential College at the University of Wisconsin–Madison. He received his baccalaureate degree from Wisconsin and his M.Phil. and doctoral degrees from Yale University, where he taught for more than a decade. Cronon, who also holds a D.Phil. from Oxford University, has been a Rhodes Scholar, Danforth Fellow, and MacArthur Fellow.

MINDY THOMPSON FULLILOVE, M.D. is a research psychiatrist at the New York State Psychiatric Institute and associate professor of clinical psychiatry and public health at Columbia University. She received a baccalaureate degree in history from Bryn Mawr College, a master's in nutrition from the Institute on Human Nutrition, and her M.D. from the College of Physicians and Surgeons of Columbia University. Her psychiatric training at New York Hospital–Westchester and Montefiore Hospital included specialties in family therapy and community psychiatry. Dr. Fullilove currently serves on the National Community Preventive Services Task Force, which will produce the *Community Preventive Services Guide* in July, 2000. She serves on the editorial boards of the *American Journal of Psychology* and the *Journal of Sex Research.* Dr. Fullilove's research has focused on the health problems of minority communities, and her current research projects examine the role of spirituality in recovery from addiction. Her book *The House of Joshua: Meditations on Family and Place* will be published this year by the University of Nebraska Press.

ROBERT FULLILOVE, III is associate dean for community and minority affairs and associate professor of clinical public health in sociomedical sciences at the Joseph L.

Mailman School of Public Health of Columbia University. After receiving a baccalau-reate degree from Colgate University, Fullilove earned a master's degree in instructional technology from Syracuse and a doctorate from Teachers College, Columbia University. Currently, he directs the masters program in health promotion and disease prevention at Columbia, where he also co-directs the Community Research Group. His research has focused on the impact of treatment programs on the lives of men and women addicted to crack cocaine, and he also has extensive experience in designing programs to improve mathematics and science education. In 1995, Fullilove was appointed to the Board on Health Promotion and Disease Prevention of the Institute of Medicine. He also serves on the Advisory Committee on HIV and STD Prevention for the U.S. Centers for Disease Control and Prevention. In 1998, he was named a visiting Falk Fellow (along with his wife, Mindy Thompson Fullilove, M.D.) at the University of Pittsburgh Graduate School of Public Health.

IRA HARKAVY is associate vice president and director of the Center for Community Partnerships at the University of Pennsylvania. He has served the university as assistant to the president, vice dean of the School of Arts and Sciences, and executive director of the Program for Assessing and Revitalizing the Social Sciences. Harkavy teaches in the departments of urban studies, city and regional planning, and history. He has long experience working to involve colleges and universities in democratic partnerships with local schools and their communities—a notable example being the West Philadelphia Improvement Corps (WEPIC), a thirteen-year partnership to create university-assisted schools. Within the Center for Community Partnerships, he has helped develop ser-vice learning and academically based community service courses as well as participatory action research projects that involve students and faculty from across the university. On a national level, he has helped many other colleges and universities to engage in this new pedagogy. Harkavy is executive editor of *Universities and Community Schools* and also serves on the editorial board of *Non-Profit Voluntary Service Quarterly*. His baccalaureate and doctoral degrees, in history, are from the University of Pennsylvania.

RICHARD P. KEELING, M.D. is director of University Health Services and profes-sor of medicine at the University of Wisconsin–Madison. He serves as executive editor of the *Journal of American College Health* and has been president of the Society for the Scientific Study of Sexuality, the American College Health Association (ACHA), and the International Society for AIDS Education. He is a member of the National Committee on Partnerships for Children's Health, and since 1985 he has served as the chair of ACHA's task force on HIV disease. With Helene Gayle, M.D. and other col-laborators, Keeling published the first studies of HIV seroprevalence among college students, reporting on research for which he had served as principal investigator. He is the author of numerous books, chapters, articles, abstracts, editorials, and videotapes concerning health issues. A hematologist, Keeling's undergraduate degree is in English from the University of Virginia, and he did his medical training at Tufts University School of Medicine. In addition to directing a complex, comprehensive health program for the University of Wisconsin and training medical students, Keeling teaches undergraduates and is active in the Chadbourne Residential College, part of the university's "Pathways to Excellence" program.

SHEILA MC CLEAR is director of special projects in the office of the president at San Francisco State University, and she has also directed the university's office of public affairs. McClear serves on the university Advisory Board for the Romberg Tiburon Center for Environmental Studies and on the advisory board for the university's Presidential Scholars program. She has taught writing and literature at the University of Hawaii and the University of Maryland, European Division.

PATSY REED retired this year after five years as chancellor of the University of North Carolina–Asheville, capping a career in higher education that included positions of academic leadership at Northern Arizona University, including interim president and vice president for academic affairs, and at Idaho State University. Reed's areas of scholarship are nutrition and biochemistry. She is the author of a nutrition textbook and holds (with her husband, a medicinal chemist) two German patents for antibiotics. Her degrees, including a doctorate in biological sciences, are from the University of Texas–Austin. Dr. Reed has served as a consultant on the transition of higher education in a market economy at the University of Lodz, Poland. In the United States, she has served on the North Central Association of Colleges and Schools' Accreditation Review Council and was a member of the Commission for the Southern Association of Colleges and Schools.

DANIEL ROMER is a senior research fellow at the University of Pennsylvania's Annenberg Public Policy Center, where he studies the influence of the media on public health and politics, as well as conducting research to identify strategies for health education among urban adolescents, with a particular emphasis on HIV prevention. Also, he co-teaches an undergraduate, academically based service-learning course, which focuses on strategies to reduce ethnic and cultural tensions, using the University of Pennsylvania as a source for case studies. Romer received his doctoral degree in social psychology from the University of Illinois at Chicago.

REFERENCES

LEARNING FOR OUR COMMON HEALTH

Burns, Wm. David. 1997. *Summary of principal findings from the 1996 Survey of Presidents and Chief Academic Officers.* Washington, D.C.: Association of American Colleges and Universities.

Farmer, Paul. 1992. *AIDS and accusation: Haiti and the geography of blame.* Berkeley: University of California Press, 16.

Gergen, Kenneth J. 1991. *The saturated self: Dilemmas of identity in contemporary life.* New York: BasicBooks.

Oakeshott, Michael. 1991. On being conservative, in *Rationalism in politics and other essays.* Indianapolis: Liberty Fund, 411-12.

Porter, Roy. 1997. *The greatest benefit to mankind: A medical history of humanity.* New York: W.W. Norton & Co., 7.

Whitehead, Alfred North. 1961. *Alfred North Whitehead: An anthology* (Selected by F.S.C. Northup and Mason W. Gross). New York: The Macmillan Company, 107.

SERVICE LEARNING AND HIV/AIDS PREVENTION: PROSPECTS FOR AN INTEGRATED STRATEGY

Barber, Benjamin R. 1992. *An aristocracy of everyone: The politics of education and the future of America.* New York: Oxford University Press.

Benson, Lee & Ira Harkavy. 1995, November. *School and Community in the Global Society: A Neo-Deweyan Theory of Community Problem-Solving,* Paper presented at the National Conference on Community Service and University-Assisted Community Schools, University of Pennsylvania.

Boyer, Ernest. 1994. Creating the new American college. *Chronicle of Higher Education,* March 9, A48.

Centers for Disease Control. 1996a. *Update: Mortality attributable to HIV infection among persons aged 25-44 years—United States, 1994. MMWR*, 45, 121-125.

Centers for Disease Control. 1996b. *AIDS associated with injecting drug use—United States, 1995. MMWR*, 45, 392-398.

Dewey, John. 1990. *How we think*. New York: DC Heath.

Dewey, John. 1927. *The public and its problems*. Denver, CO: Allan Swallow.

DiClemente, Ralph J. Ed. 1992. *Adolescents and AIDS*. Newbury Park, CA: Sage Press.

Furco, A. 1994. A conceptual framework for the institutionalization of youth service programs in primary and secondary education. *Journal of Adolescence*, 17, 395-409.

Gilman, Daniel Coit. 1969. *University problems in the United States*. New York: Garret. (Originally published in 1898.)

Harkavy, Ira & John L. Puckett. 1991. Toward effective university-public school partnerships: An analysis of a contemporary model. *Teachers College Record*, 92, 556-581.

Harkavy, Ira & John L. Puckett. 1992. Universities and inner cities. *Planning for Higher Education*, 20, 27-33.

Karabelnik, Lisa & Jeffrey Gold. 1994. *Students teaching AIDS to students. Training Manual.*

Reston, VA: American Medical Student Association.

Leslie, Stuart W. 1993. *The cold war and American science: The military-industrial-academic complex at MIT and Stanford*. New York: Columbia University Press.

Liu, Goodwin. 1996. Origins, evolution and progress: Reflections on a movement. *Metropolitan Universities*, 7, 25-38.

Markus, Gregory B., Jeffrey P.F. Howard, & David C. King. 1993. Integrating community service and classroom instruction enhances learning: Results from an experiment.
Educational Evaluation and Policy Analysis, 15, 410-419.

Price, James Robertson & John S. Martello. 1996. Naming and framing service learning: Taxonomy and four levels of value. *Metropolitan Universities*, 7, 11-23.

Porter, Judith R. & Lisa B. Schwartz. 1993. Experiential service-based learning: An
integrated HIV/AIDS education model for college campuses. *Teaching Sociology*, 21,
409-415.

Romer, Daniel & Ira Harkavy. 1996. *Evaluation of the Pennsylvania Service Scholars
Program: 1996.* Philadelphia: University of Pennsylvania.

Romer, Daniel, & Robert Hornik. C. 1992. HIV education for youth: The importance
of social consensus in behavior change. *AIDS Care*, 4, 285-303.

Smith, Albert H. 1907. *The writings of Benjamin Franklin.* New York: Macmillan.

Smith, John W. 1993. *The spirit of American philosophy.* (Revised edition.) Albany:
SUNY Press. Sommerfeld, Meg. 1996. Beyond the ivory tower. *Education Week*,
April 24, 33-36.

Struzick, Tom. 1996. *Personal communication. (*School of Public Health and the
WEPIC Replication at the University of Alabama at Birmingham.)

LEARNING ABOUT HIV/AIDS AND ETHICS IN A LIBERAL DEMOCRACY

Bell, Nora. 1991. Ethical Issues in AIDS education, in *AIDS and Ethics* (ed. F.
Reamer). New York: Columbia University Press, 128-154.

Gutmann, A. 1987. *Democratic education.* Princeton: Princeton University Press.

Keiger, N. & J. Lashof, 1988. AIDS, Policy analysis, and the electorate: The role of
schools of public health. *American Journal of Public Health*, 80: 4, 416-418.

Prashad, V. 1999. *The temper of citizenry. teaching matters.* Trinity College, 113-127.

Reamer, Frederic. 1983. The free will-determinism debate and social work. *Social Service Review*, 57: 4, 626-644.

PLACING HIV/AIDS IN PERSPECTIVE: A QUESTION OF HISTORY

Dalton, H.L. 1989. AIDS in blackface. *Daedalus*, 118(3), 212.

Fullilove, M.T. 1998 Comment: Abandoning race as a variable in public health research—an idea whose time has come. *American Journal of Public Health*, 188, 1297.

Fullilove, M.T., E.A. Lown, & R.E. Fullilove. 1992. Crack 'hos and skeezers: Traumatic experiences of women crack users. *Journal of Sex Research*, 29, 275-287.

Fullilove, M.T., R.E. Fullilove, K. Haynes, & S. Gross. 1990. Black women and AIDS prevention: A view toward understanding the gender rules. *The Journal of Sex Research*, 27, 47-64.

Mann, J.M. & D.J.M. Tarantoloa. 1998. The global picture. *Scientific American*, 279, 83.

Thomas, S.B. & S.C. Quinn. 1991. The Tuskegee Syphilis Study, 1932-1972: Implications for HIV education and AIDS risk education programs in the Black community. *American Journal of Public Health*, 81, 1498-1504.

Turner, P.A. 1993. *I heard it through the grapevine.* Los Angeles, CA: University of California Press.

PHOTO IDENTIFICATION AND CREDITS

Page ii   Human erythrocytes, red blood cells
Visuals Unlimited, °Michael C. Webb

2   HIV in lymphocyte (TEM, x80,000)
Visuals Unlimited, °Hans Gelderblom

22   Peritoneal macrophage and lymphocytes (SEM)
Visuals Unlimited, °E. Shelton, D. Fawcett

34   Vibrio cholerae (Cholera pathogen) (SEM, x1,200)
Visuals Unlimited, °Veronica Burmeister

54   Red Blood Cells (SEM)
Visuals Unlimited, °David M. Phillips

76   White blood cell leaving blood vessel, attracted by an infection/foreign or abnormal or aged cell
Visuals Unlimited, °David M. Phillips

96   HIV entering a cell (x100,000)
Visuals Unlimited, °Hans Gelderblom

106   Human Immuno-deficiency Virus (TEM, x130,000)
Visuals Unlimited, °David M. Phillips

120   HIV-1 (TEM; x240,000)
Visuals Unlimited, °Hans Gelderblom

132   Human T Lymphocyte (TEM, x18,000)
Visuals Unlimited, °David M. Phillips

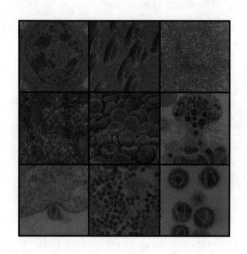